MAKE ME PRETTY, MAKE ME LAUGH

MAKEUP TIPS, INAPPROPRIATE JOKES, AND INSIDE STORIES FROM THE BEAUTY INDUSTRY

JEREMY BETH MICHAELS

D1573285

MAKE ME PRETTY, MAKE ME LAUGH

MAKEUP TIPS, INAPPROPRIATE JOKES, AND INSIDE STORIES FROM THE BEAUTY INDUSTRY

JEREMY BETH MICHAELS

Cover design, book design and illustrations by Joshua Michaels.

ISBN: 978-1-54398-471-2

28 27 26 25 24 23 22 21 20 19   1 2 3 4 5

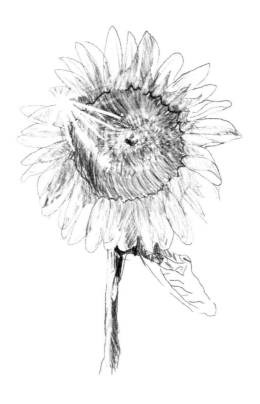

This book is dedicated to Giselle Ayala in loving memory

CONTENTS

FOREWORD

I've known Jeremy for at least 10 years. We did stand up together. She saved my life once (and not just by forbidding me to wear some horrific blush). She's rode shotgun with me through too many Tinder hook ups, a volatile marriage, a few relapses, a suicide attempt, an arrest, a divorce, a criminal trial and a heartbreak. She's not just funny, ridiculously knowledgeable about make up/skin care and extremely short but a good and loyal friend.

Jeremy did some kick ass make up for the only photo shoot of mine that I've ever liked. (I think she's a wizard.) She taught me that I DO need to moisturize my greasy skin. Who fucking knew???

As an only child raised by my father, I knew nothing about skin care or make up. And who wants to read a Kevin Aucoin book on cocaine? Not I.

She helped me prevent wrinkles as I, to everybody's astonishment, survived into my 40's with a brutal drug addiction.

I needed the basics: help with my adult acne, how to look glowy and young, how to wash my face, what masks to use besides Halloween ones. Jeremy has been my goto for all of it. Straightforward, kind, funny as hell and loving, she's taught me everything I need to snare the boys and make the other cougars jealous.

This book is great if you have ADD, like to laugh or are lazy. It's the shit we should all already know but most of us don't. It's the stuff you're too embarrassed to ask the salesgirl at Sephora when you're over 15. It's the stuff you wanna know without watching an annoying chattering chick on a Youtube tutorial. It's the info that dermatologists charge $150/hour for.

She taught me that I could wear a tinted moisturizer if I was creeped out by foundation but still wanted to rock my "junkie semi-homeless" look…in a more runway chic kind of way.

Beauty is serious business but thanks to Jeremy it doesn't have to be daunting or confusing. Now I know what's bullshit and what's effective and I've gotten to laugh while I learned about it. Jeremy is my guru for anything to do with make up and skin care and now she can be yours too.

She also told me I have very greasy eyelids (great for not aging, bad for eye liner) and that my eyes are quite close together. Jews unite!

Enjoy my beauties!

Best,

AMY DRESNER

Author of *My Fair Junkie: A memoir of getting dirty and staying clean*

ABOUT THE AUTHOR

As a beauty expert and stand-up comedian, Jeremy has spent the last fifteen years making people pretty by day and making them laugh by night. She lives in Los Angeles with her husband, adorable stepdaughter, and dachshund, Charlie.

TESTIMONIALS

In this book, just like in life, Jeremy delivers short, concise, and gut-punch funny insights into a world she knows best. I never went through an experimental stage in college, but I might now: Just so Jeremy can make me pretty. Also, I kinda wanna wear a dress.

— JEFF KREISLER, best-selling author of *Get Rich Cheating*

Jeremy Beth is literally every woman (No offense, Whitney). She's the girl that makes make-up simple by infusing her humor with expertise. She's the girl you want to go to brunch with. She's the girl you can workout with and make fun of the bobble-headed Barbie with at the same time. She's funny, down to earth, and has been through some incredibly challenging and scary life circumstances that have only added to her fierce, comedic repertoire. This book will make you laugh, help you learn, and — most importantly — make you feel pretty.

— SANDY STEC, comedian, radio personality star at 101.3 SF and KOST 103.5 LA

They say, "True Beauty Comes From Within" but what happens when you get dumped right before your father passes away from a two-year battle with cancer and you have to put your career on hold to help your mother run the family business? You put on some fuckin makeup, that's what. And if it wasn't for Jeremy Beth Michaels, and her ability to properly consult me and my problematic skin, I know I would not be able to look back at the pictures from that time and say, "Well, at least I looked great!" Every girl needs a helping hand (and some eye cream) when they're going through all that life can throw at you and I'm certain Jeremy Beth is the perfect person to be that missing link in your life.

— MARCELLA AGUELLO, stand-up comedian

Jeremy is hilarious. When I ask her about my face she tells me that if I keep my skin moisturized, I will have no problem getting laid well into my sixties. I'm a bit of a slob, and am very intimidated by makeup and beauty stores. But after meeting Jeremy, I find myself reaching out to her, asking questions about what products to get for my aging face. She's nonjudgmental, extremely knowledgeable, and very very funny. Her approach and expression of beauty help a lot of people who don't know where to begin and are afraid to ask.

— AMBER TOZER, author of *Sober Stick Figure*

Jeremy made me pretty by teaching me the benefits of good skin care while making me piss my pants with laughter.

— STEVE KASSAJIKIAN, global Urban Decay makeup artist

Who knew a comedian would know so much about skin care and beauty? I may have breakthrough formulas, but Jeremy gets astonishing laughs.

— PETER THOMAS ROTH, owner/founder of Peter Thomas Roth Clinical Skin Care

Jeremy taught me how to apply bronzer correctly and tells me I have beautiful skin every time I see her. These are two of many reasons I continue to invite her to all of my parties.

— SHELBY STOCKTON, stand-up comedian

INTRODUCTION

THIS BOOK IS A COLLECTION OF INSIDER STORIES: some pretty, some ugly, some hilarious, and some that are sprinkled with a heartfelt message or two. After each story, you'll be rewarded with a get-you-gorgeous beauty tip. Years of working in the beauty industry has shown me people generally have the same questions and concerns about beauty, but are too afraid to ask.

I've had to be a psychic, therapist and a best friend — all while doing someone's cat eye. I'm not going to lie, I can't help you with whatever other issues you might have: relationship disasters or a shitty job. But what I do know is the world of skin care and makeup. I'm the friend you connect with when you want to look your absolute best.

Did you know beauty is the only industry that doesn't decline in a recession? People may not be able to make their car payment on time, but they can usually shell out seven bucks for a new lipstick. And lucky for you, I've tried almost every product out there — some with massive allergic reactions and others with swimming success.

Now I know shopping for makeup can be intimidating. Not everyone has the patience to search through a sea of products. And maybe you don't want to feel stupid asking some snooty woman at the Chanel counter what a fucking primer is and why you need it. Well, I've talked to that bitch, and I've been that bitch, and if I have to say, "Is there anything else I can help you with?" one more time, I may implode. But here, in this book, I'm happy to share my knowledge with all you.

Besides tips, you'll get a bird's eye view of what happens behind the makeup counter. It's not all eye shadow, lipsticks, and contours; it's also dealing with the public. That's probably the best and the worst thing about the job, because all you guys are STRAIGHT UP FREAKS! No offense, but please take a chill pill. You're all wearing me out.

My experience starts waaaaaaaay back at the Sephora Call Center in San Francisco in 2000, when Sephora wasn't yet a household name. I was fortunate to learn all about fragrances, makeup, and skin care from some top international beauty educators. That same year, I began doing stand-up comedy and my life seriously started being all about lipsticks and jokes. In 2002, I packed my makeup bag, notebook, and self-esteem and moved to Los Angeles, where I've been beautifying the masses and dropping inappropriate hilarity ever since.

Being a stand-up comedian and makeup artist, I get asked the same two questions all the time: "Can you make me laugh?" and "Can you make me pretty?" Well, I can do both. My two professions complement each other, like yin and yang, because in beauty we try to conceal your imperfections, while in comedy we try and magnify the flaws. (I know I'm getting pretty deep here but when you find that perfect lipstick it's pretty close to a spiritual awakening.)

So if you want to know how to create a smoldering smoky eye, or just release a few endorphins laughing at my expense, then read on, my beauties… All you need to do is keep your mind and makeup bag open.

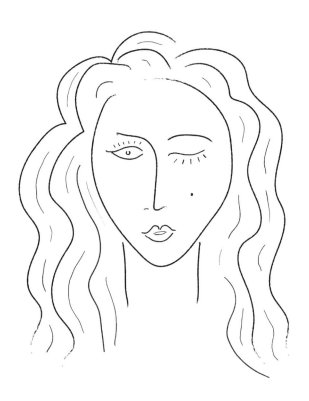

1

CLEANLINESS IS NEXT TO GODLINESS
(OR AT THE VERY LEAST USE A LITTLE PURELL)

BEING IN THE BEAUTY BUSINESS FOR OVER A DECADE, I've worked with some highly colorful makeup artists. We're a strange, motley crew but somehow we have a magical ability to make any woman spend hundreds of dollars on a whole new makeup regime just by saying, "You look really pretty."

There are some eccentric characters in the business and there's an especially interesting one that I encounter a lot. Her name is Tonya. She's a successful freelance makeup artist but what dumbfounds me is that she always looks like she just wrestled with a cat in a trashcan — and lost. Everything she seems to come into contact with sticks to her…literally. She's like human flypaper. It's not uncommon for her clothes to feature a combination of dog hair, cat hair, maybe even some bunny hair. (Yep, she has a fucking bunny.) And I'm guessing she had a spinach frittata for breakfast because she's wearing half of it. It did look delicious though.

Her hair looks like a brush hasn't graced it in about 13 years, and that's being generous. Even if you ignore her Medusa-like hair, she just doesn't look ready for "work." Perhaps you need another cup of coffee to wake you up, sweetie, and a quick sponge bath? Or how about a few rides in the Lint-O-Whirl? If that's not homeless chic enough for you, Tonya rarely wears undergarments: no bra, no underwear — nothing. I don't even go commando at home, let alone at work. Seriously, who goes to work without underwear on, unless you're a hooker? Actually, I think even hookers wear underwear. (Crotchless panties are still undies, people.) And how do I know this, you ask? Because I've been lucky enough to accidentally see Tonya's nether regions more times than anyone who's not banging her should.

One time I was forced to take a ride in her car and you know that show Hoarders? Well, her car is Hoarders On Wheels. Thanks for trying to clear an inch of space for me to sit amongst all of your crap, Tonya. And truth be told, I think that's when I had my first panic attack.

Another banner moment for me was when I saw her actually blow on a client's eyes to try to dry their liquid eyeliner. Personally, if someone did that to me I would freak the fuck out. I'm actually freaking out right now just thinking about it. But somehow she gets away with it because she's so good at what she does. Tonya has done work for tons of magazines, movies, and commercials — and the jobs continue to roll in. I guess with some creative types you just have to accept the fact they didn't learn the difference between good blowing and bad blowing. I think we can all agree that this is DEFINITELY bad blowing.

My point is, makeup artists work with the public. We get all up in your grill. It's an unspoken rule (or at least it should be) that showers are kinda cool, as is washing your hands, especially when you're touching people's faces all day long for God's sake! Tonya's fingernails are dirty and black — not the black that's cool and edgy in a Goth sort of way but in an "I don't ever want to hold your hand… ever" sort of way. So my advice to her and other estheticians is to (a) bring some Altoids because breath that could kill cattle is never cool (b) use some Purell, and (c) take a shower because yesterday's shower won't keep you clean today.

MAKEUP TIP #1

ONLY GOT FIVE MINUTES? I GOT YOU COVERED

WHAT YOU'LL NEED:

TINTED MOISTURIZER

EYE CREAM

CONCEALER

WHITE, OFF-WHITE, OR BEIGE EYELINER

WHITE, CHAMPAGNE, OR ANY LIGHT, PEARL-FINISH EYE SHADOW

BLUSH

MASCARA

LIP GLOSS

CLEAN UNDIES

Alarm didn't go off? Late night? In a rush for your nine o'clock meeting? Sometimes things don't go as planned and you have five minutes to pull it together. These nine little items will save your ass and you don't even have to thank me later.

I'll presume you've had at least 10 seconds to wash your face and put clean underwear on. Once you do that, apply a thin layer of tinted moisturizer. You can use one of the new CC (color correcting) or BB (beauty balm) moisturizers. These are lightly tinted moisturizers with extra skin care benefits. Nowadays, almost every cosmetic brand has one: you just have to pick your favorite. They help even out your complexion, conceal any flaws, and hydrate, plus some contain sunscreen to protect your skin.

Next up is the eye area. This is where your late nights will inevitably show the most but who cares? You had fun, didn't you? Pick your favorite eye cream and apply underneath your eye. Let it soak in. After your under-eye is hydrated, you can apply your concealer. Concealer hides any dark circles and evens out any discoloration. You can also apply concealer to your eyelid as an eye shadow base or to even out any redness.

To help give the illusion that you haven't actually been out until 3am on a Tuesday, take a white, off-white, or pinky-beige colored eyeliner pencil and apply it directly in your bottom (and top, if you dare) waterline. This brightens your eye area by making the whites of your eyes seem bigger, and thus a fake nap is had. If you want something a little subtler, take a pearl or champagne shimmer colored eye shadow and lightly press it onto the top lash line. When in a rush, apply a few coats of black or black/brown mascara to your top lashes only. This enlarges the look of the eyes and brightens your overall look.

Next, take some blush. Use either a rosy-pink or peachy-coral color and gently sweep it on the apples of your cheeks then blend upwards towards your outer eye. This diffuses the color so it looks natural, giving you a fresh look — even if you're still half-in-the-bag.

Lastly, tie the whole look together with your favorite champagne/beige or pinky-nude colored lip gloss. Now, you're ready to run to work, your probation officer, or wherever the hell you need to be! Just remember to wear undergarments.

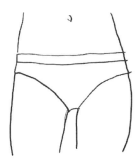

2

FOUNDATION ISN'T YOUR SKIN CARE

NEWSFLASH: FOUNDATION IS NOT SKIN CARE! Sure, you can spackle foundation all over your face and try to camouflage what's really going on. However, if all you see are zits, dry patches, and redness when you take it off, you may want to consider adopting a good skin care regimen. Foundation doesn't keep your skin balanced; it just tries to hide the fact it's out of whack — and usually fails.

When customers come in covered in a thick base, I feel like saying, "Hey, Miss, that's foundation, not cupcake frosting. You shouldn't need a spatula to apply it. And if you do, you're doing it wrong! But wait a second! Is that vanilla bean frosting? Because you do look absolutely delicious! Oh, wait. It's not?

Case in point: One day a young girl (I'll call her Buttercream), maybe 15 years old, came in with her mom. They were attending one of my facial makeover events because her mom wanted to get her daughter a product that would cover her acne. Not only did Buttercream come in wearing tons of foundation but it was also the wrong color for her. She looked ashy, which is never hot, unless you're into dead people. (For the record, I've got nothing against necrophiliacs. Fly your freak flag high — it's just not my thing.)

There's an art to getting the right color foundation for your skin. Most of us have different undertones. You want to find out if yours is olive, golden, pink, or neutral. This is crucial because whatever undertone you have is going to determine what will work the best with your skin color. You can color swab your cheek or neck area with three different shades of foundation and see which one matches the best; usually the right color will blend perfectly, while shades that don't match will be easy to spot.

Once you get the right color, you won't look like you're wearing foundation because it will match your skin tone perfectly. The whole point of foundation is to create a flawless and seamless canvas for any other makeup you apply. I see women and young girls day after day that have acute acne, lots of redness, and/or super dry or very oily complexions. When problem skin erupts, they want to cover it up. Let's sweep it all under the liquid foundation rug because if you can't see it, it's not there, right? But denial is only a river in Egypt. The problem is there, and we still see it. Sure, putting crappy foundation on is a temporary solution to cover up poor skin — but let's attack the real issue by addressing your skin type and figuring out how to take care of it.

Do some research and buy the products that are right for you. And remember, it's your face so stop being so freakin' cheap! Take the plunge. Trust me, it's worth the investment. When you go into a beauty retailer it's important to speak with a qualified beauty ambassador who knows how to treat your specific skin issue. If your skin is really problematic, you may want to consult a dermatologist. Just remember, we're all going to break out from time to time but if it's constant and you can't seem to get it under control with a good skin care regimen, seeing a professional is really your best bet.

Back to our story… I asked Buttercream if I could take off her makeup so we could get the right color foundation as well as see what the heck was going on with her face. I'm not exaggerating when I say it took about 15 minutes just to get down to her naked skin. But once her face was clean and bare, I wasn't surprised she wanted to hide it. This poor girl had a crop of whiteheads strewn along her cheeks, chin, and nose that were about a minute away from erupting on me. I wanted to give her a hug.

It was hard to see what a pretty girl she was because her skin was so red and inflamed. Bad skin is heartbreaking for women but especially for young girls who are striving to fit in with their peers. Having shitty skin can make the most confident girl turn into a timid damsel in beauty distress — and we don't want that, now, do we? So I politely asked Buttercream what she used for skin care, unsure if I really wanted to know. "You mean, like, what foundation do I wear?" she said. "No, what do you use to wash your face before you go to bed at night?" I clarified. "Oh. I just use soap and water," she said. "What kind of soap?" I pried. "Irish spring," she said. "I love how clean it smells."

What the fuck? Seriously? Now, my husband uses Irish Spring and he does smell delicious, but even he doesn't use it on his face. Well, maybe he does, but that's only because he's a dude. What do they know about skin care anyway? OK, to be fair, there are tons of guys who use delectable creams and lotions on their faces but sadly most of them don't date women.

Buttercream saw the horror on my face when she told me her soap choice. Shrugging, she quickly added, "It's what all my friends use." What I heard was, "Come on, lady. Cut me some slack — I'm only 15. All I know about is Fortnite, selfies, and Arianna Grande." I wanted to physically shake her and say, "Are you nuts? It's your face for Christ's sake." But I composed myself and said, "Listen, little blossom, I'm going to get you a couple things to repair your skin." She nodded and looked at me wide-eyed with an adolescent glimmer of hope. And that's when I knew this kid could really go places because I knew she was going to listen to me.

For her, I selected a mild facial wash — something that would clean her skin but not strip it of its natural moisture. In her case, something that has cucumber or chamomile in it would be mild enough for everyday use, but also strong enough to clean out them pores. (I turn hillbilly sometimes.) Then, I applied an oil-free moisturizer. Buttercream explained that she usually avoided any type of moisturizer because she thought it would make her break out more. Yikes! This is a makeup artist's nightmare. Never put makeup on a bone dry or unclean face — just like you don't paint a house without priming it first. I hydrated and prepped her skin with a makeup primer, which would ensure that her makeup stayed on all day. Makeup primer also evens out your skin tone and fills in any rough texture. This is a perfect step before applying any foundation. For Buttercream, we settled on an oil-free, liquid foundation with medium coverage.

And guess what? Because we properly treated her skin, I only needed to apply one layer of foundation, not 17. As a result of doing just a few "pre-steps," I needed to use much less foundation. I finished her off with a little translucent powder to absorb any excess oil and to set her makeup. Not to brag, but Buttercream's skin looked fresh, even, and not as if her liver was failing. Buttercream and her mom hugged me, both amazed at how good she looked. With foundation, less is definitely more. (The only time more is better is when it involves the carat size of diamonds.)

Now that we had set Buttercream up and running on her new beauty routine, her skin had sprung back to life. They left happy and I felt like a beauty superhero, saving one beautiful damsel at a time!

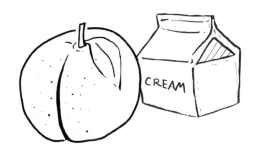

MAKEUP TIP #2

GETTING TO KNOW YOUR SKIN TYPE

WHAT YOU'LL NEED TO DO:

CHOOSE A SKIN CARE ROUTINE FOR YOUR PARTICULAR SKIN TYPE AND CONCERNS

You only get one face. So when you want your skin to look its best, heed this advice: If you treat yourself like shit, you'll inevitably look like shit. Hopefully you haven't been sleeping under a rock, or even a couple double cheeseburgers, for too long to realize that your lifestyle choices contribute to crappy skin. Unfortunately, waffle fries from Jack in the Box isn't considered "clean eating." Not drinking enough water can deplete your skin of hydration. (Wait, don't Diet Cokes and Mai Tai's count? It's a liquid!) And just because you want to rock-n-roll all night doesn't mean your skin wants to. It's a long way to the top if you want to rock-n-rock but a slooooooow and boring Baroque drop to the bottom when you look in the mirror and you've aged 20 years in two days. You may be able to skate by for a while but the truth always comes out at some point: Your skin doesn't lie. I know, it totally blows.

The good news is, if you make the time to take care of your health today, you'll be setting yourself up to look your best later in life. For example, the simple act of sleeping does wonders for our skin. They don't call it "beauty sleep" for nothing. And always and I mean AL-WAYS remember to wash your face before you go to bed. I've heard in my travels and teachings from other skin care gurus that every night you don't wash your face can age your skin up to two weeks. What the fuck is right! Even if you're extremely busy or just super lazy, at least get those face wipes and make sure no traces of makeup are left before you lay your pretty little head to sleep. In short, try and eat sensibly, drink plenty of water, and get enough sleep because achieving beautiful, balanced skin is the best preparation for your foundation and makeup when you want to look flawless.

First up, you need to figure out what skin type you actually have, rather than assuming or guessing. I can't tell you how many times I hear, "I'm sensitive." Well, maybe if you weren't using products that are totally wrong for your skin type, your skin wouldn't be so red and pissed off. Try talking to a beauty expert or esthetician that can analyze your skin properly and recommend the right products to address your particular concerns. Yes, quality skin care products can cost an arm and about four really awesome contour palettes — but they're worth it. Trust me, you'll notice a difference in your skin almost immediately.

Remember that whenever you try a new skin care regimen, your skin may freak out. It's true and it sucks but here in beauty land we call it the "honeymoon period" and it's your skin's way of getting adjusted to any new regimen. (Kinda like a new marriage — right, honey?) Even though some breakouts may occur, try sticking with any new product for at least 28 days, barring you get no serious irritation. This is the time it takes for your skin cells to naturally turn over, revealing newer, more vibrant skin. That way you can really reap the benefits of your products and see if they actually work for you. If you find that you get severe reactions, or your skin doesn't look the way you had hoped, then by all means stop using them and return them. (No, retailers don't care if you return used products so don't feel weird about taking them back. Check their return policy, but usually you will have up to 30 days to exchange your purchases with a receipt.) Once you find your skin's perfect prescription you won't want or need to use so much makeup because your natural beauty will be able to shine through. Even if you're a total bitch on the inside.

People usually fall into one of these five categories and you will too unless you're an alien: Normal, Oily, Dry, Sensitive, Combination, and one that I added for funzies: Texture. I'll also address Acne and finish with some common questions for all skin types.

NORMAL SKIN

Can you use any product and have little to no reactions? Then you're normal AF. When you have a normal skin type, you're lucky because you can cherry pick what products work best for you, making it pretty easy to compile a skin care routine. It's best to find products that don't make your skin feel tight, but not greasy either. Make sure you have a cleanser, serum, and moisturizer but be careful with peels and other treatment products. Definitely don't over-use them, or over-exfoliate your face, as this can cause the skin to get irritated. Experiment and see what works best for you.

OILY SKIN

Can you fry an egg on your face because it's so greasy? Do you have a hard time controlling shine? If your skin is oily, congratulations! You're genetically predisposed to having less wrinkles later in life than your dry-skinned counterparts. The only downside is you'll need to find products that control oil and shine. While frying food on your face might be considered a delicacy in other countries, here in the U.S. of A, we like to be supple, hydrated, and not look like a steak is sizzling on our foreheads. But fear not, pizza face, we can still get it under control with a few select products.

BREAKING BEAUTY NEWS! Just because you're oily doesn't mean you don't need a moisturizer. You absolutely do! This is one of the most common misconceptions people have in regards to their oily skin. But guess what? If you don't moisturize your face, your skin freaks out and actually produces more oil, creating more unbalance, acne, and uneven skin tone and texture issues. I know it sounds pretty counterintuitive to moisturize oily skin, but the key to beautiful skin is keeping it in balance. Something with aloe or chamomile works really nicely because it calms any inflammation from breakouts but still hydrates the skin.

You can also try using a moisturizer in gel form. Anything that has a gel-like texture doesn't usually contain any oil, so these products are your best bet when trying to control shine but also keep your skin perfectly hydrated. If you're extremely oily, or even just get oily during the day around 3pm, then an oil-free, mattifying moisturizer should be your go-to. It wondrously absorbs any oil and keeps you shine-free all day.

Once you get the right moisturizer for your skin you can start to address some other issues that come with being oily or acne prone. Unfortunately, you can be oily in your thirties, forties, or fifties and still have your skin breakout like a raging hormonal teenager. Yet just remember: the oilier you are, the less wrinkles you'll have later. So while you can't really enjoy this backhanded blessing now (Fuck you, genetics), you might be able to later, when you're 50 and still look 35. I personally wouldn't know: I make the desert look wet because I'm so dry.

You'll want to get a face wash that removes all traces of makeup and grime without stripping your skin of natural oils. Nowadays there are about five billion different types of washes out there. How do you pick? Well, the common test is, if your skin feels really tight after you wash your face then that wash is too drying for you, while if you feel like an oil slick after washing, try using a sudsy-type wash or something less moisturizing.

Using a wash with beta-hydroxyl acid is great because it really gets into the pores and cleans out all the junk that creates blemishes. It will exfoliate as well, helping to reveal newer, fresher skin.

I also like to throw in some type of exfoliation a few times a week for every skin type, including oily. Not only does exfoliating slough off the dead layer of skin but it also helps other treatment products to penetrate your skin better. (Yes, I said penetrate, you kinky freaks.) This is important when you're using specific treatment products to control breakouts. Just don't over-exfoliate because that can spread bacteria and make your skin worse.

DRY SKIN

Let's go to the opposite side of the spectrum now, shall we? Does your face constantly feel tight or do you suffer from flaking? Does your skin sometimes look dull and lifeless? Are you actually dead? If you answer yes to any of these, sorry snakeskin face but you're dry and probably look older without even trying. This is great if you're trying to use a fake ID but not so great if you don't want to be called "Ma'am" before your time. The trick with dry skin is to get products that adequately hydrate and moisturize the skin.

Use a cleanser that removes any residual makeup and leaves your skin feeling supple and hydrated, but never tight. A milk, cream, or oil-based cleanser is best because it's mild and doesn't strip the skin of natural oils. Try using one that has alpha-hydroxyl acid. This will do the same thing as an exfoliant but is geared more for dryer skin.

It's important — dare I say crucial — to hydrate your skin after you wash. This helps skin retain its moisture and protects it from the environment. Get a moisturizer that has extra hydrating ingredients, such as hyaluronic acid or shea butter, aloe, or coconut oil. You can also use a hydrating toner or skin softening lotion to really lock in the moisture after washing.

Some people like a skin regime to take two hours. (Maybe you're a Real Housewife on Bravo, or you're Korean. Man, Koreans really love their skin care.) Other people want to do it in two to three steps and be out the door. Either way, if you have dry skin, don't skip a hydrating serum. And If you do have time for an extra step, it's important to exfoliate dehydrated skin — or you won't get the best results.

The key thing to remember when you have dry skin is to look for the ingredients that deal with your particular hydration issue. Are you in the sun all day? Then pick something with Vitamin C. Do you smoke (which is so 1994 anyway)? At least move on to vaping if you must, and use something on your face that oxygenates the skin and brings back vitality and youthful glow. Hyaluronic acid is a key ingredient due to the fact one molecule holds a thousand times its weight in water so it holds hydration in the skin, helping you look supple and younger. Look for ingredients like coconut oil, vitamin E, squalane (usually made from olives), ceramides, and shea butter. Once you nail down your concern, you can get the right products that will help maintain the last bit of youth you have left. Also, make sure to protect yourself from the sun. (I know I seem like a nag about sunscreen but you should apply that shit daily.)

SENSITIVE SKIN

OK so you're not oily or dry but your skin doesn't seem to respond well to many products. Do you break out in hives anytime you try something new? Does your skin get red or do your eyes water when applying any new creams? Do you just need a hug? Dealing with sensitive skin is challenging because of the multiple ingredients in products but mild, fragrance-free products will usually work best. Also, if you know you have sensitivities to a specific ingredient, then by all means, stay the hell away from it.

For instance, one time my family and I went raspberry picking when I was like four or five and I ate so many of those tiny hot pink gems that I got a severe allergic reaction. My lips swelled up so much I was the laughing stock of our family for like two whole days. Looking back, I resembled any LA girl in her mid-twenties to mid-thirties with their lips overblown with Juvaderm. I guess I could get a bucket of raspberries and find out if it still happens, making it possible for me to fit right in with all these other clowns in Los Angeles. The point is, now I know raspberries make me swell up, I'm not going to buy any skin products that contain real raspberries unless I want to look like an asshole. By the way, rarely have I ever seen a natural looking lip job. You're not fooling anyone, sweet (HUGE) lips.

Even when you're sensitive you still need to properly cleanse the skin. Choose a mild, foaming or cream-type cleanser with soothing ingredients like cucumber, aloe, rose, oatmeal, and chamomile. This type of cleanser will gently remove makeup and dirt without irritating the skin. Never over exfoliate when you have sensitive skin as this may cause redness and inflammation. If you have severe redness, eczema, or cystic acne, those soothing ingredients will really help. Getting your skin in balance will be a little tougher for you, but totally doable. The key is finding that ingredient that works to calm your skin, while also addressing any of your other concerns.

Weird thing is, even if you have sensitive skin you can still be oily in some areas and really dry in others. Make sure to hydrate and calm the skin while still trying to attain balance. I usually suggest an oil-free hydrating serum and moisturizer because this helps retain hydration without causing any irritation.

COMBINATION SKIN

(IT'S LIKE THE BI−SEXUAL OF SKIN TYPES)

Are you oily in some places but dry in others? Bitch, you are complicated! Surprisingly, having combination skin is the easiest to maintain. You can use different products to treat the different areas of your face. If you have an oily T-ZONE area (across your forehead and down your nose), use an oil-free or mattifying product in that area only. You can add extra hydration by using moisturizers and serums only where you need it.

When picking out a moisturizer for combination skin, look for something that has a whipped-like texture. When it's whipped it's lighter in density than some of the heavier creams but will do a great job hydrating the skin, while not creating future havoc for the oilier parts of your face. Using a lightweight, oil free moisturizer with hyaluronic acid is your best bet.

TEXTURE ISSUES

Does your skin have a crater-like feel or appearance? Does your skin appear bumpy or rough to the touch? Does your face look like you need a steamroller to smooth out all that shit? Are your pores bigger than you'd like, and still show through when wearing a full face of thick foundation? Then, I'm sorry to say, you most likely have some texture issues.

Friends and clients ask me all the time how they can smooth out their skin. It's really painful to see a teenager or someone even older with texture issues. It looks rough and if you have that Mars-like look to your skin and you're not an astronaut, then you'll probably want to add some more advanced treatments into your skin care routine. Resurfacing the skin takes time and consistency, but after you pick out a cleanser, serum, and moisturizer that work, you should try a chemical or physical exfoliation, and retinols. When you exfoliate you get rid of any dead cells, allowing newer healthier cells to come to the surface. This also helps brighten your complexion and will help smooth out any rough texture by turning over older cells. Retinols help diminish hyperpigmentation, reduce fine lines, and treat acne and scars. You can also go the pro route and schedule an appointment with an esthetician if you aren't getting the results you want with over-the-counter products.

ACNE

Do you have over-productive hormones? Unfortunately, this can create unsightly bumps on our skin — at any age. It's not fun to have acne in your teens and twenties, let alone in your thirties and forties. The good news is if you have visible breakouts bumps and/or redness, you can use topical acne spot treatments and masks to prevent future breakouts. Make sure to use a sunscreen during the day when using these products because some acne ingredients, like salicylic acid and retinols, make your skin sensitive to the sun. It's actually best to only use them at night.

If your breakouts are driving you nuts, I recommend doing a weekly mask. Look for ingredients such as sulfur, clay, charcoal, and pumpkin because they'll help draw out impurities and clear bacteria from clogged pores. But just warning you: save your sulfur products for when you're home alone watching The Notebook because sulfur smells like a jock's underwear.

Trust me here: use it solo. Or use it when you don't want to get laid. If you've always wanted to cock block yourself, then use sulfur on your face and wear socks with sandals. You'll probably never get lucky again. Table for one, forever!

If you're consistent with your mask, you should start to see results pretty quickly. For some oilier skin types, only certain areas tend to break out so the new thing the kids are doing is called multi-masking. It's using specific masks for particular areas of your face. If you have some areas that are dry and yet some that are oily, use the mask for acne directly on your breakouts or congestion, and use a hydrating mask where you tend to be drier. That way you are multi-tasking while you are multi-masking. (Yep, I just wrote that. Deal. I'm a real douche sometimes.)

FOR ALL SKIN TYPES

Here are three questions I get asked, oh, about ten times every hour: What are the benefits of exfoliating? Do I have to use a toner? Do I really need to buy an expensive serum? Don't worry, none of these steps are mandatory but your skin will look WAY better if you do them. No pressure, right?

WHAT ARE THE BENEFITS OF EXFOLIATING?

Exfoliating reveals a newer you and all skin types can benefit. It can be done two ways: chemically or physically. Chemical exfoliation is when you use an actual acid or enzyme to do the sloughing. Physical is when you have to manually exfoliate with your hands or an electronic brush, such as a Clarasonic, or those other weird ones carried in Sephora that basically look like vibrators. Who the fuck are we kidding here? I'll take three! And put on some Prince, you sexy motherfucker!

The best types of physical exfoliation use rice, jojoba beads, almonds, walnuts, or anything somewhat grainy. Make sure the "beads" are complete spheres otherwise they actually end up nicking your skin over time and you don't want to ruin your only good selfie side. And please steer away from any sort of plastic micro beads, which are now banned in some countries because they create havoc in our oceans, lakes, and rivers. These synthetic beads absorb toxins in the water and are then eaten by marine life; if we eat any fish, we run the risk of ingesting the toxins as well. But because exfoliation is crucial in revealing newer, fresher skin, the key is to be environmentally conscious when picking out your next product. If it's not good for all the fish or mermaids in the sea, it's definitely not good enough for me. (I'll pass on sushi for a while anyway).

Either a physical or chemical exfoliation product will help to control acne, decrease pore size, diminish fine lines and wrinkles, scars and also help to fade any redness and age spots. It's like a magic eraser for your face. Choose the one that's best for your skin type and skin sensitivity and I suggest doing it weekly. Exfoliating is an important step in your routine because when you don't, your treatment products have a harder time seeping into the deeper layers of the skin to give you all the amazing benefits you're looking for. So, in essence, you're risking throwing away your hard earned money if you don't get that dead layer of skin off.

DO I HAVE TO USE A TONER?

I get asked a lot about the benefits of using a toner and if they're necessary. It's really a personal preference. Using a toner after you wash will close the pores but you can do the same thing by splashing cold water on your face. Closing the pores is important because you prevent pollutants or dirt, which can cause inflammation and breakouts, from getting in your skin. You can also get treatment toners that address different skin concerns, such as a hydrating, firming, mattifying, or exfoliating. It just depends on the results your trying to achieve.

DO I REALLY NEED TO BUY AN EXPENSIVE SERUM?

Serums aren't cheap, sweetie. But they are one of the most crucial must-have products in your skin care routine when it comes to changing or improving your skin. Luckily, there's a serum for every type of skin concern so everyone wins. Yay! Serums have the highest concentration of active ingredients so they should be one of your key purchases, especially when you're looking for visible results. Choose the texture that feels best on your skin. Some have a watery, oily, milky, or creamy texture, while others have a viscous, gel-like texture. It's really a personal preference on formula but because serums are thinner and have a lower or smaller molecular weight, they're able to be quickly absorbed into the skin, letting you really reap the benefits of the product. All it takes is a good skin evaluation from a professional to see what your skin needs the most. Since I'm dry and my skin can look dull at times I'll use a Vitamin C serum (for brightening) and then follow it with a hyaluronic serum (for hydration) during the day. If you have more than one concern like me, considering using two serums at a time. Just make sure the serums you choose are suitable for day or night. Some night serums will make your skin sensitive to the sun, especially if you're using an acne or retinol serum.

BONUS TIP: When using multiple serums, always follow this rule: apply the thinnest (watery) to thickest (more viscous). This way, the more watery of the two will seep into the skin effortlessly, while the thicker one will lock in all that moisture and other skin-loving ingredients — so you can look as plump and juicy as Kim Kardashian's fake ass.

FOR A GOOD TIME FOLLOW:
@JEREMYTHEGIRL

BEAUTY SHOPPING LIST

- ☑ WHITE + BLACK TEA
- ☑ ROSE
- ☑ CUCUMBER
- ☑ CAFFEINE
- ☑ ALGAE
- ☑ HYALURONIC ACID
- ☑ PEPTIDES + NEUROPEPTIDES
- ☑ CERAMIDES

3

DOES THIS FACIAL EXPRESSION MAKE ME LOOK HUMAN?

A YOUNG GIRL CAME TO ONE OF MY EVENTS and asked me in all seriousness to help her pick out some wrinkle cream. I thought she was buying a gift for her mother, grandmother, or great-grandmother until she confessed that it was actually for her. Wait, what? First of all, she said she was only 14. Second of all, she was only 14 for cryin' out loud!

At this point, I wasn't sure if I should be angry at the world or sad for this already insecure young girl. She barely had any boobs and here she was, just on the verge of hitting puberty, already worried about wrinkles? Shouldn't boob worry come before wrinkle worry? Shouldn't you have to be old enough to order the senior special before you start worrying about looking like the senior special?

Could she really have wrinkles that were worth blowing off hanging with her boy-crazy friends to catch a ride with her mom to the mall? Her mom told me the girl had been begging for something to fix her (invisible) wrinkles for the last three weeks. She said this while eyeing her daughter in a very disapproving manner, recounting that the daughter had also told her she wanted to get cheek implants and Botox. That day, the girl's mom said she could get some "special creams" for her "wrinkles" but this was really maternal code for "no fucking way" on the implants or Botox. Under no circumstances was she allowed to get any type of cosmetic procedures done until she was an adult or a stripper — whichever comes first.

I know from experience that girls are bombarded with negative messages about their appearance from the moment they play with their first Barbie. Barbie, with her eternally frozen perfect face and an impossible-to-attain body, only teaches girls how to be unrealistic about their looks from the very beginning of their impressionable young lives. Then you have fashion magazines, YouTube videos, Instagram, selfies, and billboards besieging these girls about how the "perfect" girl should look and that no girl should ever age. And if they do, they better find a way to hide it.

I asked myself, Is this really what teens are concerned with these days? Isn't there a teen fuck-up-du-jour they can snapchat about? When I was 14, I was drinking shitty Bartles & James peach wine coolers while smoking Djarum cloves and trying to sneak out of my parents' house with my girlfriends. Probably to go make out with some boy I definitely shouldn't be making out with. What can I say, growing up in San Jose, California, was wild. In truth, I didn't start worrying about wrinkles until about two hours ago and it's been the longest 120 minutes of my life.

Living in Los Angeles really skews people's views of reality. You wouldn't find this fear of aging in say, Nebraska, where teens are too busy fighting juvenile diabetes and building storm shelters. But here on the West Coast, we have it so easy because all of our worries are embarrassingly superficial. The two dreaded questions in Los Angeles are "Do I look fat?" and "Do I look old?" And this is before teens are old enough to know what getting old or fat is supposed to even look like.

In many societies, age is not condemned: it's revered. Older people are respected and considered wise. They've earned every single one of those wrinkles through the ups and downs of a long and hopefully interesting life — they're battle scars. Many things, like cheese or wine, get better with age and you'd think people would want to think the same about themselves. But women are not supposed to age. At all. At least not here in Los Angeles.

You might as well pickle everyone here in LA. Youth reigns supreme and even over 40-year-olds are shopping at Forever 21. In LA, I see young girls dressing like they're realtors or corporate bankers just to look older, even dyeing their hair gray, and then I spot older women dressing like Britney Spears circa '98. I'm talking middle-aged women sporting a half shirt, insanely short skirt and pigtails. These women claim to abhor ageism yet they're playing right into it. Oops, we all did it again.

Personally, I feel that it's irresponsible to give this message to younger girls. It instills a fear of maturing. You see that line there? Well, it's a smile line. Imagine that! Traces of joy! You know how they say 40 is the new 30? And Tuesday is the new Thursday? And Orange is the New Black? Well, facial expression is the new dead. Doesn't this worry anybody else?

To the young LA girl I said: "You don't need to worry about your face right now. The lines that will come eventually are from smiling or crying. It's called emoting and it means you're not dead inside." I told her to go get into some trouble. "Go post something inappropriate and take that provocative half-clothed selfie with the stupid duck face. Go live your life. Enjoy your youth. If you're below 50, eat sorta healthy, get a bit of exercise, cool it on the crack smoking and you'll be just fine."

I refused the opportunity to sell her some wrinkle cream for her invisible lines and, as she walked out, she turned around and stuck her tongue out at me. At least now she's acting her age, I thought. I refrained from telling her that when you stick out your tongue like that for too long it causes you to get those wrinkles around your mouth that look like a cat's asshole. Meow, bitch!

MAKEUP TIP #3

LOOKING YOUTHFUL, NATURALLY

WHAT YOU'LL NEED:

MOISTURIZER — ANY LIGHT DAILY MOISTURIZER WITH SPF

A FOUNDATION BRUSH, BEAUTYBLENDER (SPONGE SOLD AT MOST RETAILERS),
OR YOUR HANDS (PLEASE WASH THEM FIRST)

AN ILLUMINATING OR HIGHLIGHTING CREAM (ONE WITH A SOFT CHAMPAGNE,
BRONZE, OR PINK IRIDESCENT WORKS BEST)

EYE CREAM

SUNSCREEN

If Cher says she can't turn back time, then what the hell am I supposed to do? Actually, there is something. For a nice dewy, youthful glow, mix a little illuminating highlighting cream (a pea size amount) with your moisturizer or foundation. Apply the mixture as you would any other foundation, with either a foundation brush, Beautyblender, or your fingers. Using a brush or Beauty Blender provides a more polished look but if you're in a rush, your hands will work fine. Another easy look is to apply a little bit of the illuminizer on the tops of your cheek bones, upper arch of your eyebrows, the bridge of your nose and, lastly, your Cupid's bow (the top curve of the upper lip, right above your lip line). This makes your skin look fresh as a daisy, even if you have one foot in the grave.

But makeup can only do so much. It's usually in your mid- to late thirties when all those late nights and bad choices start to show up on your face so your late twenties are a good time to start being conscious of the anti-aging products that are out on the market. Eye cream can come sooner, while sunscreen should be compulsory for people of any age. Have you heard that saying, "A sunscreen today saves nine fine lines later?" Neither have I, because I just made it up. But it sounds pretty legit so let's assume it's true. Clients often say, "I don't need to wear it because I work in an office all day so I'm not even in the sun." Joke is on you, Malibu Barbie. All those office lights you sit under all day contain both UVA (aging) and UVB (burning) rays. You're getting hit even when you don't even think you are.

There are two types of sunscreen out there: chemical and physical. Chemical sunscreen gets absorbed into the skin and physical lays directly on top; they both help block spots and discoloration from getting darker or spreading, while protecting you from harmful rays and preventing premature aging. But here's the bummer: you must reapply every two to three hours. Since I was a total idiot growing up in the eighties, I would purposefully lay out in that blazing hot sun all day, chain smoking, and willfully absorbing those light daggers of cancer from the prime, peak hours of 10am to 2pm. Then again, anytime is prime time nowadays considering the earth will probably blow up any minute from global warming. (Are you sensing my positive side yet?) And I'll be damned if I don't look as hot as the earth itself on the way out! We just didn't know any better and I'm paying for it now, with these lovely, different colored patches all over my face. Had I known the importance of wearing sunscreen back then, I might have avoided premature aging. Oh well, fun in the sun yesterday, tons of fine lines tomorrow. Sigh.

BONUS TIP: I wish someone had told me this when I was 20 but… Whatever you put on your face, also put on your hands. Our hands have little to no defense from the outside world, unless you wear gloves 24/7 (and if you do, you're pretty weird anyway so maybe add a top hat and learn a couple magic tricks). Putting sunscreen on will prevent age spots from popping up later. At some point if you see some discoloration rearing its evil head on your hands, use a retinol at night and sunscreen during the day. This is the best prescription for hands that are ready to hold anything from a forty-ounce to a penis or glass of rosé: spot free.

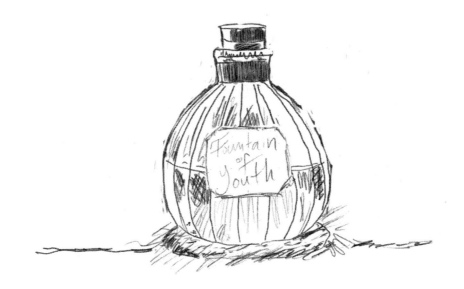

4

DON'T BE A DICK

HAVE YOU EVER BEEN AT A RESTAURANT and you see a patron being a dick to the wait staff? When that happens, it's usually over something stupid like the absence of a lemon slice in their glass of water. Calm down, asshole! Don't act like she just slapped your Grandma. She forgot the freakin' lemon.

I feel for those waiters and service people in general — they have to deal with a lot of disrespect. Likewise, people are often unnecessarily rude to me when I'm doing their makeup. Don't people realize that when you're impolite to your server or makeup artist, it's a guarantee you'll get a wad of spit in your food, or a horrifyingly surprised look to your eyebrows? And that's kind of a lose-lose for everyone.

One cosmetic company I worked for was located in a really high-end outdoor mall in Los Angeles. I would get flashed daily with black Amex cards, which always meant to me "this bitch has some money." I'll be honest: sometimes I wish that bitch was me! But alas, it wasn't.

I was usually cutting coupons and buying a huge burrito somewhere because you can split that shit into like four meals when you're scrimping with cash.

Not to brag, but I was getting paid a whopping $13.76 an hour to help the elite women of LA, who would sport Gucci belts, Dior sunglasses, Louboutin's, and diamonds easily big enough to finance a small third-world country. I had to bite my tongue because not only is the customer always right but big-ass diamonds are always more right — and I like to shine bright like a diamond just like anyone else. (You're so right, RiRi.)

One sunny day I was finishing up a woman's makeup, setting her look with some finishing powder, when she looked at me, pointed to my forehead and said, "Aww honey, you could use a little Botox. You don't want to look years older than you are, do you?" No, actually I do. In fact, the only reason I ever took up drinking, smoking, and sun tanning slathered in Banana Boat oil was to look older. Thank you for noticing. But in all seriousness, I'm 4 feet, 11 and ¾ inches tall. (You would add the three-quarters, too, if you were me.) That's short enough to still fit in a booster seat. So from the back, I actually look like a fat nine-year-old girl — light years younger than this bitch.

I gritted my teeth and said, "Well, thank you for your opinion." In my head, I continued thinking about her comment in a disturbing interior loop. I need Botox? Do I need Botox? And then I started examining myself in the mirror and a silent self-esteem breakdown ensued. Prior to this conversation, I was cool with my eternally worried expression. It made me look concerned and empathetic… forever! I don't think she was trying to be mean but rather what I like to call "Angelino Helpful."

People can be cruel in ways you wouldn't expect because they feel like you want to know their unasked-for opinion. I can barely stomach annoying "constructive" criticism from my mom. ("You really think you need that extra cookie, hun? Your pants are looking a little snug.") But as a professional I had to eat that woman's comment and silently obsess about my age on the inside. Mmmmmm… age. Of course, later on I asked all my friends if they thought I needed Botox and they said, "Hell no!" Even if my friends were lying, I don't care and that's why they're my friends and not yours.

MAKEUP TIP #4

MASKS TO LIFT YOUR FACE AND MOOD

WHAT YOU'LL NEED:

INSTANT FACELIFT MASK OR TREATMENT MASK OF YOUR CHOICE

FLAT FOUNDATION BRUSH OR FACIAL MASK BRUSH

WASHCLOTH

Q-TIPS

YOUR CLEAN HANDS

For a temporary lift, use a flat foundation brush or facial mask brush to apply a thin layer of an instant facelift mask to the areas that you want to be line-free. Once dry, these masks can leave an egg white-type film on your face but don't freak out. Just get a damp washcloth or a Q-tip and gently wipe off any white residue. You'll notice you have absolutely no lines. Pretty crazy, right? Follow with your usual foundation application and makeup then try to stop staring at yourself in your phone. Some of these facelift masks can last for as long as eight hours so have a blast but you better get home before midnight, Cinderella, or else your whole beautiful face will fall down. Tick Tock.

But masks aren't only for Halloween anymore. There are some amazing products on the market, particularly if you have a special occasion and want to look your best. Because I like to be on top of anything on my face, I do an "at home" facial every so often. Even more beneficial is to do a mask regularly, say once a week. For most masks you put them on anywhere from five to 15 minutes. Some come in saturated sheets that you apply directly to the face. Some will dry completely, some peel off, some you have to get a wet washcloth and rinse them off. There are so many to choose from but always read and follow the instructions on the label so you get the best results. Once you get in the habit of masking regularly, your face will thank you and even a newborn baby will be envious of your skin.

Masks generally come in these categories: hydrating, brightening, purifying/detoxing, exfoliating, and sleeping masks.

HYDRATING

Take a good look at your skin and see what your face needs the most. Is your skin dry or does it feel tight? If so, this mask is a good choice. If you don't hydrate your skin properly you tend to look older and your skin won't have that healthy glow. When my face looks really dry I go for ingredients like avocado, coconut, hyaluronic acid, seaweed, rose oil, or shea butter because it softens my skin and brings back some of that youthful color (which is really hard to do when you're nine million years old).

BRIGHTENING

If you feel like your skin looks dull and drab, you'll want to grab a brightening mask. These

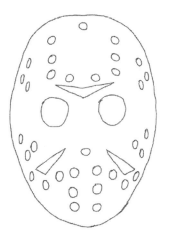

NEW: HYDRATING "JASON" SHEET MASK

HYDRATE WHILE YOU FREAK PEOPLE OUT...OUT...OUT...

PERFECT FOR FRIDAY THE 13TH!

are especially good to do if you have a special occasion because they tend to put the life back in your skin. I usually choose one with Vitamin C, which is a natural antioxidant that reduces melanin formation — you know, those pesky little sunspots that seem to sprout out of nowhere and never go away. Vitamin C helps to prevent and diminish spots while giving you back your glow. Another great type of brightening mask is oxygen-based. If the oxygen is depleted in your skin cells, usually by environmental factors, your skin won't look as luminous. Putting the oxygen back in your skin will give you a rosy, youthful glow, while plumping up any fine lines and wrinkles. It's a great pick me up, especially when you need to look your best.

PURIFYING OR DETOXING

If you're prone to oily skin, or suffer from congestion and clogged pores, get a good purifying or detoxifying mask. I usually look for ingredients like mud, clay, charcoal, or sulfur. When the skin is congested or you have visible black heads, you'll want to use one of these ingredients because they tend to have a magnetic effect in pulling out all the impurities.

EXFOLIATING

Sometimes my skin doesn't look as fresh and vibrant as I would like, and looks kinda "blah." In that case, I'll usually do a good exfoliating mask. As I previously explained, exfoliating increases your cellular turnover by helping to remove dead skin cells from the surface, revealing a fresher, newer you (almost like being a virgin… again). The ingredients you want to look for are glycolic acid, which is made from sugar, and fruit enzymes, such as pumpkin or papaya, which eat away the dead skin cells. I know that sounds like there's a skin-eating monster on your face, but it's kind of true.

SLEEPING

The best and latest craze I've seen in the beauty world is the sleeping mask. There are many on the market so pick the one that's right for you; simply apply it before bed and then you can go nighty night. And wake up looking amazing.

BONUS TIP: One beauty hack I've found on the mean streets of narcissism and in most retailers are these super convenient hydra-gel eye patches that contain loving, de-puffing, brightening, and tightening ingredients all in one product. If you want a great pre-treatment for eyes that will decrease bags, firm, and hydrate, look no further. Put these little beauts under your eyeballs for about 10 to 20 minutes while you're having your morning coffee, sexting, or pretending to listen to your conference call. After the allotted time, take the suckers off and WOW! Now you're brightened, de-puffed and de-wrinkled.

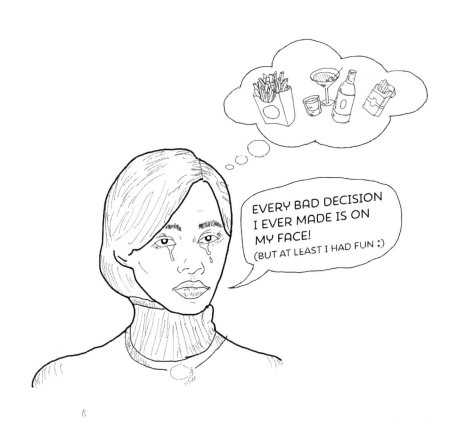

EVERY BAD DECISION I EVER MADE IS ON MY FACE!
(BUT AT LEAST I HAD FUN :)

5

EYES: THE WINDOWS TO YOUR BEAUTIFUL BLACK SOUL

I KNOW IT'S HARD TO BELIEVE the very things that allow us to see (unless you're missing both your eyes, in which case that sucks) pose the ability to show our age faster than we can say, "Resting Wrinkle Face." Our eyes are the first place we notice age on a person because this is where most of our facial expressions come through. All those years of smiling, laughing, crying, and wailing like a baby start to make their mark on the sensitive skin around our eyes, making it crinkle up whenever we express our countless, daily fucked up emotions. The delicacy of our eye area makes it really challenging to prevent and conceal the evidence of a life well lived — or not so well lived, depending on who you ask. Maybe don't ask my mom.

Some people say with pride, "I've earned every one of these lines," while others go to the extreme of trying to look as if they've never felt any emotion at all. Think of some of our beloved celebrities that went a little too far under the knife. I like to be somewhere in the middle. I'm not 20, but I'm not 70 either. I like to have a slight "worn in" look with a floaty, yet sparkly, ethereal thing going on. Basically, I want to look like any airbrushed model in an Anthropologie catalogue.

Both our physical and emotional environments affect how we age so if any area of your life causes you immense stress on the inside, you can bet it's starting to show on the outside. Lucky for you we're living in the age of "self-care." Hey, it's OK to be selfish now! Take some time for yourself to meditate, do yoga, write in your diary (which is actually a way too long Facebook post). Whatever it is that brings you some calm and peace in your daily life, do it regularly.

One of the best compliments I've ever received was that I looked "well-rested." If I could bottle that and sell it, I would. It's the look I'm constantly aiming for. And while I get irritated with the countless 17-year-olds who come in all dewy and disappointment-free asking for an eye cream to hide their crow's feet, I have to admit I admire their determination to look wrinkle-free forever. The truth is, you can only hide the challenges of your most difficult years for so long. I should know, 2003 is creeping up on me something hard, people.

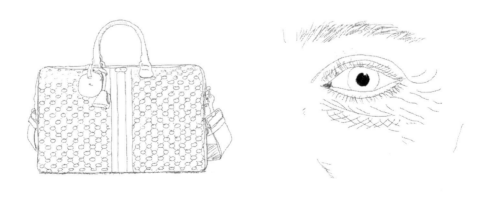

ACCEPTABLE BAGGAGE   UNACCEPTABLE BAGGAGE

MAKEUP TIP #5A

FULL CIRCLE EYE CARE

WHAT YOU'LL NEED:
EYE CREAM OR GEL
YOUR RING FINGER TO APPLY

I'm a firm believer that the only bags you should have are the kind that go in the overhead compartment of an airplane. Not under your eyes. The good news is, you can prevent premature aging by using an eye cream daily. No exceptions! Take the time now to protect this tender eye area and you'll thank yourself later. Because the under-eye area has less oil-secreting glands than the rest of your face, it's a priority to keep this area hydrated if you want to diminish and prevent the appearance of fine lines and wrinkles.

Eye creams can be expensive. They come in really small packages and when you open them up they don't sparkle at all like a princess cut diamond but just sit there being all like "cream and shit." You should still make the investment. There are two forms of eye cream: gels and creams. Gels soak in quicker than creams but creams tend to be more hydrating, which is especially great if you feel your under-eye area is on the drier side. (The only time "dry" is good is when it's describing a beautiful fine wine, amiright?) Using eye creams or gels daily will magically help to blur, hydrate, and plump up any fine lines, plus prepare the area for makeup. If you don't prep the skin, you run the risk of your makeup separating throughout the day, looking crack-y (gross), or even worse, settling in all those pesky fine lines that we're all trying so hard to hide.

If you have dark circles from untold late nights, hereditary dark circles, or dullness around the eyes, look for an eye cream that will instill some brightness. Ingredients like Vitamin K, arnica, Vitamin C, and ginseng will all do the trick. Or maybe you have under-eye bags that could hold all the 18 pairs of shoes you're bringing for your girls' trip in Vegas. In that case, the best ingredients are caffeine or cucumber, which will firm, tighten, and de-puff. Remember: even though we can cover bags with makeup, it's a good idea to get products that will help illuminate the under-eye area beforehand.

BONUS TIP: When applying an eye cream ALWAYS use your ring finger. This is our weakest finger in terms of strength so it allows the effective, gentle placement of whatever treatment you're using without pulling, tugging or — God forbid — streeeeettttttching that delicate area around the eye. Always use eye cream to hydrate and smooth out the surface before you apply your concealer.

If you start to see little white bumps around your under-eye area, you're using an eye cream that's way too rich for you. The bumps are called "milia" and they're basically cysts you can't pop. Bummer, right? So if you see these little buggers, you'll probably want to use something a little less viscous, like a hydrating gel or a lighter weight eye cream.

What happens when your eyelids start to droop? This is not one of the things your mother prepares you for. I'm actually still a little pissed about it. If you start to notice your eyelids becoming less taut and more on the crepey side (It's the worst word, right? It sounds awful and it is!), then it's time to find an eye product suitable for that upper eyelid. Some skin care lines have eye products targeted for tightening and hydrating this particular area. You may ask, "Do I really have to get two separate eye creams? One for under my eye and one for my actual freakin' eye lid?" Unfortunately, the answer is yes. As I've put on blast before, the skin below your eye is extremely delicate but so is the upper eyelid, so it's best to treat them a little differently.

If you've already spent a fortune on eye cream and find you still have visible dark circles under your eyes, try putting an orange, peach, or melon color correcting concealer under your eye before you put on your regular concealer. Just make sure to choose the right shade for your skin tone. Use a concealer brush to apply a thin layer of the color corrector and blend it in upwards underneath your eye, then follow with your usual skin tone colored concealer — and all darkness will be erased. Also, don't forget to apply concealer between the bridge of the nose and the inner corner of the eye. This area tends to be very dark on some people, as well as overlooked, so it makes a huge difference when you color correct and conceal. Once that's done, the whole eye area really brightens up and you're ready to apply your favorite eye makeup.

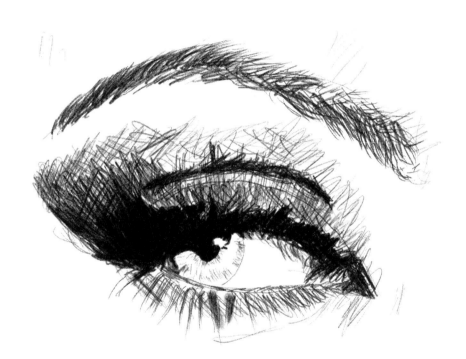

MAKEUP TIP #5B

CREATING THE PERFECT SMOKY EYE

WHAT YOU'LL NEED:

EYE SHADOW BASE OR YOUR CONCEALER

BLACK, BROWN, NAVY, OR GREY EYE SHADOW.

BLACK OR BROWN EYELINER — EITHER A PENCIL LINER, A LIQUID LINER PEN, OR CREAM IN A POT

IRIDESCENT OR HIGHLIGHTING EYE SHADOW IN PEARL, CHAMPAGNE, OR LIGHT PINK

FLAT EYE SHADOW BRUSH

SMUDGING BRUSH

CREASE/BLENDING BRUSH

THIN, POINTED TIP EYELINER BRUSH — IF USING CREAM LINER IN A POT

MASCARA

Once your eye area is prepped you can create a really gorgeous and easy smoky eye. This look is great for nighttime or any time you want to add a little vavoom!

To do this, I usually put concealer or an eye shadow base all over my eyelid, from lid to brow. This evens out any discoloration on the lid, prepares the area for eye shadow to be applied, and helps your shadow to stay put. Pick your favorite darker color eye shadow and use a flat eye shadow brush to apply it from your lash line up to just a smidge above your eyelid crease. You can get the desired intensity by gently pressing the shadow onto your lid. Then take your crease brush, which is a soft, full brush, usually dome shaped, and use it to blend out any harsh lines. Use your brush like a windshield wiper and go back and forth until completely blended.

Next, I take the same eye shadow color and place it directly under the lower lash line using a smudge brush, which has a small, stubby, firm but soft tip. This brush enables you to "smoke" or smudge your makeup out, blurring any harsh lines so the eyeshadow looks seamless and blends perfectly under the eye.

After that, it's time for eyeliner. There are three types to choose from:

PENCIL LINER: This is the best for beginners because it's easy to create different looks and experiment with different colors using a hand-held pencil. Being able to hold the pencil directly gives you maximum control when lining the upper and lower lash line, and it can easily be applied to the waterline: the inner rims of your lash line.

CREAM LINER IN A POT: This is not the easiest to use if you're a novice. It takes a little practice but once you get the hang of using a fine or flat tip brush, you can experiment with different looks and styles with the precision of a surgeon. Cream liner can be applied to the upper and lower waterline, as well as the external upper and lower lash line.

LIQUID LINER PEN: This is trickiest of the three because it dries quickly, but it's really the best option when you want your look to stay put all day and night. And lucky you, if you happen to be caught up in a category four-hurricane (That would suck, sorry!), you would still look awesome. Just have some Q-tips ready for any mistakes. I personally don't apply liquid liner to my waterline; I only use it for my upper lash line when I want a perfect winged liner.

Take your eyeliner of choice and apply it to your top and bottom waterlines; applying liner here can add darkness to a smoky eye and also brighten up tired eyes, depending on the color you use. Traces of eyeliner will probably spill from your waterline onto your skin so use the smudge brush to mesh this into your eye shadow, creating that rich, dark, smoky effect. Also use the brush to perfect any mistakes. For added drama, you can add a dark eyeliner to the top lash line after you've applied your eye shadow. Go for that slightly winged, cat-eye look by angling your eyeliner up towards your outer brow bone.

Finally, take a little iridescent eye shadow — or highlighting shadow in pearl, champagne, or light pink — and apply it directly to your brow bone, under the arch of your eyebrow. Use a flat eye shadow brush to do this and then use your blending brush to smooth it all out. Highlighting the brow completes your look and helps make the eyes pop. Finish with a few heavy coats of mascara to the top and bottom lashes. I'll usually complete my look by applying concealer under the eyes to erase any mistakes. Then even if I've colored over the lines eight hundred times, you'd never know.

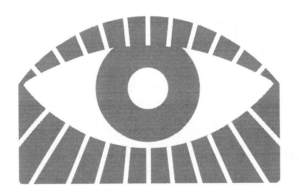

6

MOVE OVER FRIDA KAHLO: THERE'S A NEW BROW IN TOWN

A COLLEGE FRIEND OF MINE was always searching out the ultimate bargain — especially when it came to her beauty regimen. She felt that all beauty products were made from the same stuff anyway and thus she didn't need to spend more money to get the same results.

Let me preface this story by saying that she had a serious brow issue. She acquired a bad habit of tweezing her eyebrows in her early teens and after way too many self-prescribed plucking sessions, had a grand total of four eyebrow hairs left. After some research, she realized she could get her brows tattooed and would never have to worry about those pesky hairs again. Forever perfect brows!

From what I knew, permanent makeup was big in some Asian communities. I've seen brows, eyeliner, and even lip liner tattooed (Ouch!) on women, but honestly it scared the shit out of me and nobody I knew personally had ever had it done. That said, I'm all for being supportive of my friend's ideas, whether they're brilliant or stupid. The fun part is waiting to see which way it goes.

My friend found what could loosely be called a legitimate beauty school. You know the type of place that promises a full-time job after you graduate, setting you up to do makeup for Print, Film, and TV. They usually cost a fortune to attend but at least the students get to practice on actual people while getting class credits. For the client, it's much cheaper than going into a professional salon and so you'd think this would be a win-win. You'd be wrong. When you're getting your face tattooed, it's probably not the smartest idea to go to a novice. Just sayin'

Well, lo and behold, she did it anyway — of course. And guess what? They royally messed her up. One eyebrow was slightly higher than the other one and they were both thicker in some places than in others. Both eyebrows looked like caterpillars crawling on her face, which was particularly unfortunate as she had a bug phobia. When she came over to show me, it was hard to keep from laughing and to keep a straight face. I was shaking my caterpillar-free head and wondering, What the hell did you expect? Are you really surprised? You paid $29.95 and expected perfect brows from a 22-year-old who isn't certified yet? Now, I'm no genius but this screams worst idea ever!

A few months later she tried to get her tattooed brows professionally removed, which did not look like it worked. Over 10 years and a whole barrel full of concealer later, the brownish/purple sharpie-esque strips have started to fade to a low-grade grey. But let this be a lesson for anyone thinking tattooing is the best way to go: Makeup tattoos are freakin' permanent and if they happen to mess up, you'll be left looking like the love child of Frida Kahlo and Groucho Marx. Hi, sexy!

MAKEUP TIP #6

USING YOUR BROWS TO FRAME YOUR FACE

WHAT YOU'LL NEED:

ANGLED BRUSH

BROW PENCIL, OR BROW POWDER THAT COMES WITH A WAX

BROW COMB

HIGHLIGHTING POWDER FOR BROW BONE

Brows, if done right, will enhance your facial features, give you an almost non-surgical lift, and bring out your eyes. If you neglect them, you may look like a super cheap asshole that's afraid of tweezers. Think if you had some beat-up awnings on the front of your house and everything else looked amazing; the only things people would notice would be those awful, shitty awnings. Well, that's what happens when you don't keep your brows up.

Don't ever neglect them. If you can't do them yourself, it's a good idea to get your brows professionally done every couple of months either by waxing, threading, or tweezing. Once you see how pretty you look with cleaned up, well sculpted brows, you'll be amazed. Keep in mind, your brows are as individual as you are. If you like a bushier, fuller or more natural looking brow, go for it. Maybe you want a thin-ass gothic look because you love looking like a member of the Cure, or perhaps a soft angle is your more your thing. Whatever style you choose, remember the world is your eyebrow pencil.

Once your brows are in the desired shape, take your brow powder and use an angled brush to sweep across the color, making sure to tap out the excess, or use a brow pencil that matches your brow color. Gently apply the powder or pencil onto your brows in a feathery motion, filling in any bald or sparse spots, and following your natural arch. If you don't have an arch, carefully pencil or powder where you want it to be and add more as needed. Once you're done, comb out the excess color and set with the clear wax or clear brow gel. Then step back and look at yourself in the mirror. Admire how put together, polished, and awake you look.

For even greater impact, you can add some highlighting powder to your brow bone. This gives the illusion of a lift by highlighting the brow area and framing the rest of your face. Now you can stay out all night and even if you haven't slept, you'll look as if you did. Suckers!

BONUS TIP: If you have no brows at all, you can get a plastic, cut out stencil that takes the guesswork out of perfectly sculpted brows. You just have to be able to color inside the lines and hold it in one place. To be honest, I failed coloring book as a kid so this never worked for me.

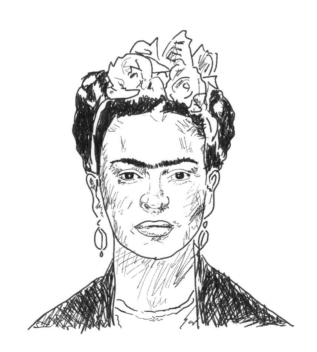

7

TO PARABEN OR NOT TO PARABEN

WHEN IT COMES TO THE BEAUTY BUSINESS, we live in a consumer savvy culture. There's a plethora of easily accessible information about beauty products and these days a lot of people want them to have organic, vegan, and cruelty free ingredients. Such products are readily available at most retailers and often pop up in the ads on social media sites. Most of the time I do believe in finding the best ingredients for things that are going in, and on, my body. (Is glitter organic?) But I have absolutely no problem using a completely synthetic or un-organic product if it promises to diminish my crow's feet.

Am I vain? Do you need to ask? Are there shards of glass or snail excrement in my eye cream? Bring it on! Oh, it has ant legs, spark plugs, and goat testicles but it's guaranteed to improve my collagen and elastin by 65% in two weeks? I'll take 47, please. And so would about 97% of the population. You better believe I'll slather almost anything all over me, like baby oil before a wrestling match in Turkey. (Wrestling is Turkey's national sport, by the way.)

One question I'm constantly asked is, "Does this have parabens in it?" For those of you who don't buy your makeup at Whole Foods, and aren't lucky enough to procure your products from a certified organic farm, parabens are a class of chemicals used primarily as preservatives to prevent bacteria and mold from forming — and they're found in about 85% of the cosmetics on the market. There's some controversy about them because parabens were deemed xenoestrogens, or agents that mimic estrogen in the body, which may affect overall estrogen levels. There are some studies that show this may lead to an elevated risk of breast cancer and reproductive issues in women.

This is where you have to decide what you put on and in your body. For me, I found in my research that the parabens in the products I choose are in such miniscule amounts that it doesn't cause me real concern. But that's my personal choice. And not to brag, but I'm a cancer survivor myself and I'm still smearing anything and everything on my face and body if it will make me look better, faster, stronger. (Thanks, Kanye.)

About 85% of all makeup contains some sort of preservative, unless you're going fully organic. Even then, there will likely be an additive to make the product stable and longer lasting. Cosmetics are usually good for a year after you open them. Without the necessary evil of one form of a preservative or another, most products would disintegrate and spoil within a week or two. Think of pasteurized milk. It's the same idea with your makeup. You don't want that eighty-dollar night cream to spoil now, do you?

It always makes me giggle when I get asked if something has parabens or preservatives in it. More often than not, the paraben-free products people are looking for are the ones that claim to banish cellulite, make you thinner, or grow your hair to Rapunzel length in just three hours — yet they're really asking if the product in question is "all natural." Yeah, lady, it's made from kelp, coffee grounds, and pipedreams.

One day, a woman with long brown hair came in weighing maybe a hundred pounds soaking wet. She was probably in her late twenties, wearing a flowy floral dress and headband, like a flower child from the 1960s that found the one working Transporter in all of greater Los Angeles. She wanted a makeover to try out some new trends but she was only interested in vegan and paraben-free products. Truthfully, I was just curious if the commune had reported her missing yet. But — and here's the kicker — she wanted something that would make her eyelashes longer.

OK, so let me get this straight, Lady Macbeth… You want some weird miracle product, currently used for glaucoma patients, which happens to grow your lashes longer, but you, in fact, don't have glaucoma and you're also willing to put it on your eyes — the only two things that enable you to see — just so you don't need to use mascara? And your main concern is that the product may contain parabens? OK, then.

She was insistent, saying, "I'm very careful about what I put on my face!" I didn't know what to say because her skin looked scaly and dry. Apparently, she had been using the "natural elements" skin care range: stuff like wind and gravel. For every item I'd suggest, she would pause, and ask, "But are there parabens in this?" I said, "Well, yes," and then gathering up my last ounce of patience, I added, "But you know what? We're all going to die anyway and soon we'll probably find out that even naps cause cancer, so you might as well look pretty as long as you can." She looked at me, grabbed her stuff (eyelash-growing product in hand), said Namaste, and left. I get it now. Great lashes trump parabens. Noted.

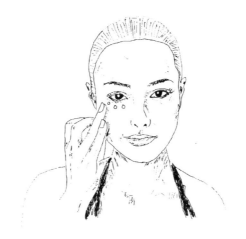

MAKEUP TIP #7A

GOING PARABEN-FREE

WHAT YOU'LL NEED:
YOUR ENTIRE MAKEUP BAG

For a lovely paraben-free look, THROW IT ALL AWAY. But if you want to be pretty, USE EVERYTHING IN IT: moisturizer, serums, eye cream, foundation, blush, eye shadow, eyeliner, mascara, lipstick, and lip gloss.

I'm kidding, you guys. Nowadays you can buy all the products you want, without all the added ingredients you don't. It is out there. Many high-end brands offer vegan, paraben- and cruelty-free products, just waiting to be picked up by you and your socially and environmentally conscious ass. However, I'm going to be pretty: parabens and all. See ya later, granola fuckers.

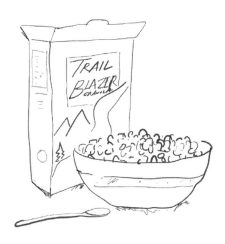

MAKEUP TIP #7B

GETTING BAT-WORTHY LASHES

WHAT YOU'LL NEED:

FALSE EYELASHES (INDIVIDUAL AND STRIP), LASH EXTENSIONS, OR LASH
GROWERS

EYELASH COMB

LASH GLUE

A PAIR OF TWEEZERS

SCISSORS

MASCARA

EYELINER

Clients often ask me if lash growers work and if they're worth the investment. They are worth it, if you're consistent. I tell people to put the treatment tube by your nightstand and apply it before you go to bed, on the top lash line only. Most brands have a product that will last one to two months. You can find a few different types at your local beauty retailer these days — just take a look at the ingredients to see if it's something you want to add to your routine. I used one about four years ago, after losing a lot of hair, and my lashes became thicker and are still fuller. They usually run at about $50 to $80 but it will really depend on the brand. You can also get a prescription but they'll cost less over the counter. Some people have had instances of discoloration either on the eyelid, or their actual iris. Freaky, right? I think the takeaway here is to use what you feel comfortable with, and remember, this is going on your eyes! If at any time you see discoloration, stop using immediately.

Another option is lash extensions. They either come in synthetic or mink. My only advice is less is more. I have a few friends that go a little cray-cray with the lashes. They are either so full that it looks like there are huge spider legs on their eyelids, or so long they could probably braid and bead them. In my humble opinion, if you're going for lash extensions, go for natural length and fullness. Otherwise, it looks way too overdone for everything other than a black-tie event or a costume party. The goal is to look like you have a generous sweep of mascara on the lashes, without the clumps. Usually, you'll have to get a refill every two to three weeks because our lashes naturally fall out. For a complete full set, it will run at about $150 to $200 and for the refill it's roughly $50 to $65. It's definitely not cheap to bat our eyes.

To me, the easiest, cheapest, and quickest non-committal way to attain beautiful lashes is by using false lashes on a strip with glue. Usually brands will have several different types, from super dramatic and full to a more natural, subtle, girl-next-door look.

Before you use the glue, place the lashes on your eye to see if you need to cut them down a bit because they're too long. If you do need to trim, cut from the outside end. Once you get the desired length, you're ready. The trick when applying lashes is to place the glue directly on the strip and wait a few seconds for the glue to get tacky before placing the strip on your top lash line. I usually start my placement in the center of my lash line and then smooth out to either side. You can perfect your placement by using an eyelash tool (usually sold with the lashes but could be sold separately), or using basic tweezers work just as well. You can also buy individual lashes and place them anywhere you want extra fullness, without using an entire strip.

After you're done applying lashes, if you see any visible gaps along your eyelid, fill them in with a little eyeliner. Finish with a few coats of mascara then take a step back, bat your lashes, and you're ready to blink on command! "Why, no, officer, I didn't know I was speeding! But I think my lashes were." Wink, wink.

Seriously, if you're looking for one thing to make yourself feel instantly glamorous, put on some eyelashes. It's the quickest way to go from boring to boomshakalaka!

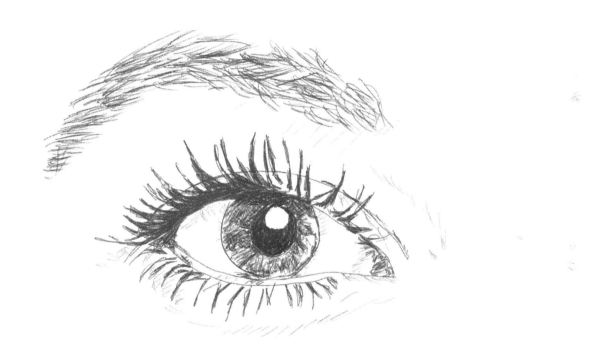

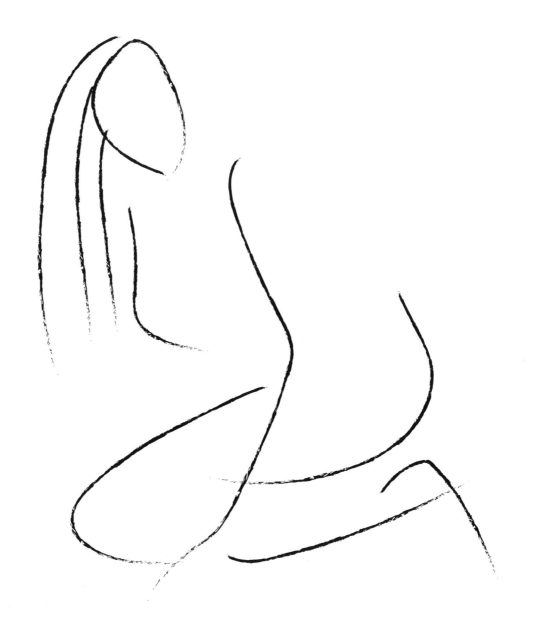

8

RIDDLE OF THE SPHINX.
OOPS! I MEAN, RIDDLE OF THE CHEEKS

I WORK IN MANY DIFFERENT COSMETIC RETAILERS all over the West Coast and one of the most affluent areas is Orange County, California. This means seeing a lot of "ladies of leisure," fake boobs, diamonds, and shitty, entitled attitudes. If my work in the OC were made into a TV show it would be called Real Extra Housewives Of Any Southern Californian City. Sometimes you get the ladies who are still chasing the leisure or the fake boobs but they already have the entitled attitude. Many women come in and spend six to eight hundred dollars on makeup without a second thought. I want to say, "Hey, lady, you just dropped my rent money on 73 eye shadows!" But I don't. I just put on some lip gloss and smile.

I always have an eye out for the women who come in late Friday or Saturday night. That timeframe is usually a bad sign as more often than not the customer has either been dumped, or is about to be dumped. What that means for me is that there's no way I'm leaving early now. It's like clockwork — just when the store is about to close and I've got plans to meet up with some friends for a much-needed after work cocktail, "Needy Nancy" comes strolling in. She'll say she wants makeup but maybe what she really needs is a long, long hug and all I want is to get the hell out of there. So I'm already annoyed because I know what's coming next...

A disheveled woman, who I'll call "Nancy," came in one night. She had no makeup on and looked like she'd been crying. I felt somehow irritated and compassionate at the same time — like when you see someone trip and fall. You feel bad for them yet you can't help but laugh. I cautiously asked, "Do you need any help finding anything?" She answered with a shrill voice, "Well, I'm trying to find a blush color. It's not like baby pink, but it's not peach either. It has some gold shimmer, but not too much shimmer because, well, you know, I'm old. I don't want to look like a stripper. But I want something that I can wear to give me a hint of color, so I don't look like a walking corpse."

She then proceeded to tell me that she didn't get the house, car, or jewelry in the divorce settlement (which is why she married him in the first place — it wasn't for love. Touching, really). And that she cheated on him, and because of her infidelity she was now solo. There would be no easy street for her. After explaining that she had never worked a day in her life, had always been supported by her parents or her many, many boyfriends, she said she really needed to catch a new man "hook, line, and sinker" to support her Orange County lifestyle — and, goddammit, she was going to do all that with blush. All I knew was that I going to be her punching bag/ therapist for at least the next hour. Fuck me!

"Well, let me pull some colors for you and we can try them on," I said. I took a deep breath then tried to get all spiritual by visualizing all my chakras clearing any negative energy and surrounding me with white light, which isn't hard to do in the fluorescent glow of the store lights. Walking up and down the aisle, I picked out every color I could find that matched her specifications, ending up with at least 35 colors to show her. We tried Blissful Berry, Aphrodisiac Apricot, and on and on, but she wasn't having any of them. One color was too light, that one too dark, this one too pink, another too shimmery, and yet another not shimmery enough.

This went on for at least an hour and nothing was working for her. It was like smelling hundreds of perfumes without taking a break; after a while they all smell the same. I started thinking maybe there should be a color called Miserable Mauve because that's what every color looked like on her.

Stranger still was that she became completely manic during my search for her perfect blush. She started staggering up and down the aisle over and over again as if she had lost her keys. Finally, I asked her, "Did you lose something?" She said, "No, but if I don't find a blush today, I don't know what I'm going to do." So I had to buckle down and dig in. We try on more. And then more. Then, out of nowhere, she started raising her voice at me. "This is too mauve and this is too brown and this is too pink!"

We just went through the entire color wheel of blush so at this point I want to throw my hands up and say, "I'm out, lady. You're on your own." But, at the end of the day, my job is customer service so you have to put up with any and all people no matter how difficult or ridiculous they may be.

I knew this lady wasn't going to find what she was looking for and I was losing whatever patience I had left. This was quite possibly my longest work shift ever and I had a party to go to and this bitch was holding me up. "You aren't helping me at all," she whined. "I thought you guys are supposed to be the experts." Then, after a long pause, she said, "I guess I'll have to go somewhere else." Never mind the 542 colors I had presented, she thought it was my fault we couldn't find the right color — nothing to do with her lack of soul.

Remaining professional, I looked at her — mildly amazed — and said, "Well, I'm sorry we couldn't find what you were looking for today. Maybe come back tomorrow when you have fresh eyes?" And that was it, she picked up the keys she kept "losing" and left. I was like, Thank you for dumping your life of indiscretions on me, along with the lingering and somewhat depressing thought that no one is faithful to anyone. Thanks for that. Then I looked around and saw I had different blushes open on every available counter. All I could say to myself was, Wow, Needy Nancy suuuuuuucks.

I could have begged her to stay, but come on… I wanted her to get the hell out of there so I could go hang out with my friends, which, by that point, I needed direly. I felt sad for her because she needed to fill a void within herself that no perfect shade of blush could ever satisfy. Pretty deep, right? Well, that's how I roll when I'm working late on a Friday. It was like trying to solve the Riddle of the Sphinx, but, for her, it was the unsolvable Riddle of the Cheeks. There would be no enlightenment for Orange County's Miserable Mauve and fuck her because I'm late for an eighties party and I have on my perfect, Patrick Nagel-esque blush. Just call me "Rio" as I'm dancing on the sand. (That's from Duran Duran if you didn't grow up in the eighties, like me.)

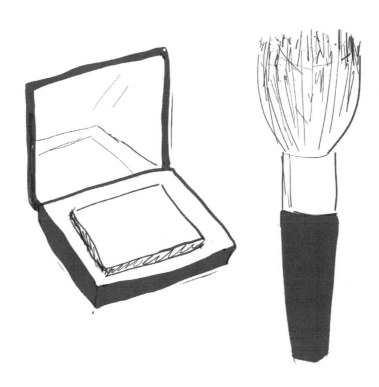

MAKEUP TIP #8

CREATING A SUN-KISSED GLOW

WHAT YOU'LL NEED:

BLUSH BRUSH

BRONZER

BLUSH COLOR OF YOUR CHOICE — YOU CAN USE A POWDER, CREAM, OR LIQUID.

To look like you've been partying in Rio, take your blush brush and sweep it across your favorite bronzer. Tap off the excess powder and use your brush to trace a backwards number three on your face. That is, start at your temple then go to your cheekbones then all the way to your chin — and repeat on the other side. This mimics where the sun would naturally hit the face, and everybody looks good with a little kiss from the sun (even if it's le soleil de L'Oreal). You learn the "backwards three" in Contouring 101. Other contouring tricks can be used to sculpt out the cheekbones you don't have, disguise a dreaded double chin, create a smaller looking nose, or define the jawline for a more chiseled look.

Now move onto your blush. There are three forms to choose from:

POWDER: My favorite and perfect for all skin types.

CREAM: Works great on drier skin, but any skin type can use it.

LIQUID: For all skin types but you have to work fast because it will dry quickly, so doing one side of your face at a time works best. I usually use my fingers for the easiest application.

Depending on what type of blush you're using, get a little on your fingers or on your brush (tapping away any excess), then smile, look at your gorgeous self in the mirror and apply the blush directly to the apples of your cheeks, with upward sweeps. This will give your cheeks just the right amount of "flush." Finish by applying some highlighter to the tops of your cheekbones, Cupid's bow, and the bridge of your nose for a beautiful glow. Not only will you look like you just came from Brazil, but you'll look like you just got laid there too.

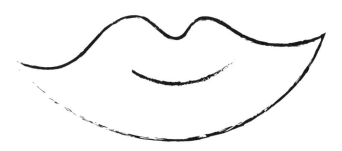

9

OUR LIPS SHOULD BE SEALED

SOMETIMES DOING A MAKEOVER CAN BE TRANSFORMATIVE, not only for the client but also for the makeup artist. Doing just a few quick tricks with color and concealer can easily take somebody from looking womp womp to YASS QUEEN! With the right amount of artificial "glow," anyone can look like they've just come back from a delightful month on a yacht called "We're Fucking Rich," while gently sailing in the Maldives with three hundred of your closest friends, drinking everything that's served with a little paper umbrella.

One day, a lady came in and thank you baby Jesus because it was a super slow day, where half my time was spent trying to look busy. So I was happy when she approached me and said she had a date that night, wanted a touch up, and to buy a few new items to add to her miniscule, tattered makeup bag. She proudly showed me all three of her existing items.

First up was a dollar-store black eyeliner that was so used, it had been reduced to a small nub. When she handed it to me, I actually thought it was a pebble. Really, lady? You can't fork out six bucks for new eyeliner? Second thing I fished out was a pukey, dusty rose lipstick. The only people who should have a dusty rose colored anything are people I don't really want to know, just sayin'. That color blows. She also had mascara that was so dried out she actually had to add a couple drops of water to it. Shredded snakeskin would've seemed moister. Nasty.

After seeing the sad contents of her bag, I sat her down and went to town. I grabbed some moisturizer, foundation, bronzer/blush, eye shadow, eyeliner, and mascara then instructed her on how to apply each item. Finally, I offered her some easy day-to-night looks.

We got to talking and I found out she was 53 and had divorced two years prior, after her ex had an affair with a 35-year-old woman. As a result, she'd had a complete breakdown, moved from Oklahoma to sunny California for a job at a computer company, and made a fresh start. I really admired her balls. I mean to break free and start over at 53 really impressed me. She was an extremely pretty and social woman: petite, blonde, very chatty but maybe a little too friendly. She asked me if I had a boyfriend and I said, "Just dating right now. Nothing serious." Then she started asking me all these personal questions about sex toys and lube and I'm not going to lie, it got a little weird. I said, "Well, we all like to get down, right?" trying to interject a little humor and deflect from this bizarre conversation.

With my mouth shut, I kept nodding and applying her makeup as she was rattling on about her new online affair with this guy she'd met on Match.com. She was going to meet him that night for the first time and wanted to look "effortless, beautiful, and gorgeous." I don't mean to brag, but I think I succeeded. As I was finishing her lipstick with a final layer of nude lip gloss, she said, "Man, my lips are so dry." I said, "They don't seem dry to me." Then she looked at me with all seriousness and said, "Not those lips." And glanced down and pointed at her groin.

At first, I didn't want to compute what she had just said. Her lips are dry, her lips are dry, kept going through my head like a news ticker. Over and over. She was talking about her fucking vagina — her fucking vagina lips! Over ten years in the business and this was definitely a first... and hopefully a last! Now, I consider myself extremely open-minded but there's a line (or a lip in this case) that must be drawn when sharing personal information with a complete stranger. She said, "Well you know, once you turn 50 it's all dry down there." Um, no, I actually hadn't thought of that golden day, but thank you for making me start to obsess about it.

It became pretty awkward after that confession. What are you supposed to say when someone discloses something like that? "Thank you so much for letting me in on this fact about you and now all I can think of is your vagina, which apparently is as moisture-free as dried chili peppers. You know, the ones that have been sitting out in the caliente sun for over 10 years, which you have to soak for three days just to get somewhat hydrated again." Bon appetít!

The thing about working with the public is that you have to put on an act sometimes, like, "This is old-hat to me, honey. I've been privy to this type of insider information for a while now." So I said, "Well, I'm sure chemists have come up with tons of stuff for that. Like, there's Viagra for the guys." What do you talk about after that? As you can imagine it was pretty silent. But I starting thinking, there's got to be something for ladies who have that "not so wet" feeling, not to be confused with the "not so fresh" feeling. And in fact, you can find remedies for both these problems at a pharmacy — but, please, not the beauty store!

Truth be told, I could do without thinking, feeling, or smelling any of these concepts for the rest of my natural born life. I smiled tightly as I finished her face then grabbed her chosen items and sent her on her… uh… dehydrated way to the register. Once she was out of earshot, the other girls on the floor who had heard her comment rushed over to me. We all looked at each other and burst out laughing. I'm not sure if we were laughing because it was so gross, or out of fear because we, too, will be old one day and our lips — either set — will be dry AF like hers.

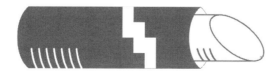

MAKEUP TIP #9

DIY LIP EXFOLIATOR

WHAT YOU'LL NEED:
OLIVE, JOJOBA, OR APRICOT KERNEL OIL

TEASPOON OF ANY SUGAR (WHITE, BROWN, COCONUT)

WATER AND A WASHCLOTH

NUDE COLORED LIP LINER

NUDE COLORED LIPSTICK

CHAMPAGNE COLORED LIP GLOSS

Do you feel like your lips (on your goddamn face) are dry? Is your kisser not in tip-top shape? Loose lips sink ships but dry lips suck. Here's a little home remedy I do once a month. I get a teaspoon of sugar and some olive oil. If you want to get really fabulous, some apricot kernel oil is nice too. Mix these two together, grab some with a spoon, place it on your lips, and gently rub for a minute to exfoliate. Don't swallow the mixture — not because it will kill you but because it tastes like shit. (Trust me, I've tried it.) Wipe off the concoction with lukewarm water and a washcloth. Notice all your dry, dead skin has gone.

Next, take a nude colored lip liner and outline your lips then fill them in. Apply your favorite nude color lipstick and follow with a slightly shimmery champagne lip gloss, just in the center. This will create a fuller look to your lip. And voila! Your lips are now ready for whatever love comes your way! And it's moisturized!

10

SNAP, CRACKLE, AND POP!

MANY MAKEUP ARTISTS REPRESENT A VARIETY OF BEAUTY BRANDS. It's standard practice to interchange between a skin care line and a makeup line — so we're well versed in both. Sometimes we team up with each other and do a facial and makeover event, which is what we were doing on one unforgettable occasion.

It was pure luck — bad luck — that my co-workers gave me the first customer of the day. And let me tell you, Ms. First Customer was not what I was expecting. She didn't know we were doing the event in the front of the store, even though there were floor-to-ceiling windows with posters and signs. That bothered her because she didn't want anyone looking at her while she was getting a facial. OK, lady, I can understand a little privacy, but you're not a celebrity and I don't see the paparazzi congregating, so calm the fuck down, pretty please.

She also let me know she was thirsty… and cold… and did anyone have a sweater… and, "Is there any goddamn heat in this building?" Then it happened. She sat down and I got a close look at her skin. Gasping internally, I took a deep breath and stared at the plethora of growths that covered a third of her face. Of course, I stayed all smiles — I'm a professional, after all — but I was a little speechless. Awwwww man. I kinda felt sorry for myself. I had to give her a facial. I didn't want to be rude but all I was thinking was, What the hell is all over your face, lady? Then I realized, they're skin tags! WTF is right. They literally looked like Rice Krispy's hanging from every viable inch of her face. At any moment I felt as if I was going to hear Snap, Crackle, and Pop!

Thankfully, nobody spilled any milk on her so that didn't happen. But I was still trying to block out the fact that her face was coming at me in 3D. I'm sure I stored it all away for some terrifying future acid flashback. (Ahh, the subconscious brain — never a dull moment. Seriously, I can't wait.) But now I know why she didn't want to be seen. Who could blame her? I guess I was the one that needed to calm the fuck down and be more compassionate. Yet I couldn't help wondering: If you happen to have things hanging off your face, why not go to a dermatologist? No one should be OK with that shit. Why hadn't she done anything about it?

But I started feeling bad for her. And I wanted to help her. So I pretended her skin was completely normal and I think she appreciated it. I really wanted to give her the most incredible facial where, when we finished, her skin would somehow be model-perfect and she would weep with happiness, tip me profusely, and skip out of our event to newer, skin tag-free pastures. Maybe I was having an acid flashback.

What I learned while doing the facial is that her name was Karen. She was a volunteer for Alzheimer patients and she lived with, and took care of, her elderly grandmother. Yeah, I felt like a total dick after I learned all that too. It was a great lesson for me and really for all of us. This woman was a fucking saint. She was so busy taking care of everyone else in her life that she didn't have time to take care of herself. She told me this was the first time she'd ever had a facial. Ever. I held back some tears and decided I would try my hardest to never pass judgment on someone's looks again. In a world where the outside seems to be valued way more than what's inside, I didn't want to perpetuate the stereotype.

I ended up doing a super luxurious gold anti-aging mask and a moisturizing hand treatment. I also applied some gel eye treatments to really pamper her before she went on to our makeup artist. She deserved it. When Karen got up from this 20-minute escape from reality, she thanked me for being so kind and said this was the first time she'd been so relaxed in months. I may have gone into the situation a total asshole, but I think at the end of it I came out half a prick.

I realized that one of the best things about working in the beauty industry is being able to make someone feel pampered, special, and pretty — especially when they need it the most. And believe me, I totally get it: I have this really long, wiry black neck hair that somehow manages to grow three feet in an hour. (Wanna sleep over?) I keep a good watch on my face, too, for any visible growths, scarring, discoloration, loss of firmness, etc. The good news is there are treatments for almost every type of skin condition and concern these days.

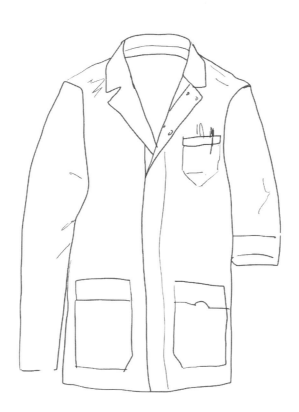

MAKEUP TIP #10

TREATMENTS FOR WHEN YOU NEED TO GO PRO

Sometimes we need a little help from someone in a white lab coat. If you have skin tags, acne scars, pit marks, deep wrinkles, discoloration, uneven skin tone, or loss of firmness and you find the treatments available at your local makeup mecca aren't cutting it, you may want to schedule an appointment with a dermatologist, esthetician or a doctor. This is especially true if you're looking for visible results.

These are some of the best treatments I've found:

MICRODERMABRASION

This treatment is good for uneven skin tone, fine lines, and wrinkles, acne, age spots, light scarring, sun damage, and clogged pores. So pretty much everyone. Microdermabrasion involves "sandblasting" or spraying the skin with abrasive microscopic crystals. This process removes the outermost layer of dry, dead skin cells to reveal younger, supple, healthier looking skin. Even though it sounds kinda creepy, it's really effective. This treatment might cost anywhere from $75 to $200, depending on the place. Results can last anywhere from six months to a year, depending on how well you treat your skin after the treatment. Personally, I really like doing these about once a year. It can be a little uncomfortable and can feel like an emery board being brushed across your face (Sounds pretty comfy, right?) but the results are definitely worth the money. It's like you shave about five years off. Like, literally. Or at least it feels like it. Ouch! But then you look in the mirror and it's all, Ooh la la.

DERMABRASION

If you need a more aggressive treatment for your skin because of deep scars from acne, previous accidents or surgeries, or you're merely concerned about fine lines and wrinkles, dermabrasion may be a great option. With dermabrasion, the surgeon scrapes away the outermost layer of skin with a rough wire brush, or a burr containing diamond particles attached to a motorized handle. This scraping is done down to the safest level of skin to help minimize and diminish visible scars and wrinkles. Yikes, is right. The treatment is done in a doctor's office and, depending on the severity of your skin condition, you could be put under anesthesia. The average price for this is around $1,000. If the skin is severely damaged, you may need multiple treatments to get the desired result. I particularly recommend this for anyone who has experienced extensive scarring due to acne, and none of the over-the-counter treatments have worked.

However, there's some downtime you need to be prepared for. You probably won't be able to go to work for a couple weeks. Your skin will be red and quite sensitive. There could be some tingling sensations and you could have some problems eating due to swelling. (When I hear that part, I'm like, I can't eat? Then I'm OUT! I'll live with my jacked-up skin and eat at Home Town Buffet forever, thank you very much.) But honestly, this treatment is for someone who has serious texture issues. We're talking like the scumbag mean dude named Craterface in the movie classic, Grease. You remember that guy? If not, look him up.

I had a friend who had skin just like that. He tried everything. Went to all the dermatologists. He did the juice cleanses to purify from within and shit. He used this lotion and that potion, changed his diet, and drank more water. Every recommendation that came his way he tried with even more conviction. Nothing worked. So he decided he would try dermabrasion as his last resort. He coughed up that moola and I'm happy to say he wasn't disappointed. In fact, we were both shocked at how good the results were.

After about a month of strictly following the doctor's orders while being bright red, sensitive, and basically looking like a cherry lollipop with eyeballs, we eventually had a "skin layer reveal party" to celebrate. I mean, what else do you do when you live in LA and work in cosmetics? You celebrate that shit. This treatment is not for the meek or broke. But totally worth it if you want do it.

IPL

Another great treatment is IPL, or Intense Pulse Light. This is ideal for age spots, sun damage, and visible dilated blood vessels. The treatment uses a bright light combined with specific filters that end up filtering out wavelengths, except those taken up by pigment and blood vessels. This light then penetrates below the skin's surface, damaging discolored pigment (melanin) and visible blood vessels. The skin naturally heals itself by removing the damaged tissue and, as a result, newer, smoother, more even toned skin is revealed. The best thing about this treatment is that there's essentially no down time.

IPL has been described as feeling like someone is snapping rubber bands on your face but at least it's usually quick. If you have severe sun or age spots, it may require more than one appointment and sometimes discoloration will look worse before it gets better. Just be patient. It usually looks amazing in a couple weeks. The usual price for one treatment is anywhere between $150 and $350. Usually people with a lot of discoloration will need about three to five treatments to see real results. Another plus about IPL treatments is that it also helps to boost and stimulate collagen production. The only downside is that it doesn't help with wrinkles but it will help with firmness and tone, as well as pigmentation.

SKIN TAG REMOVAL

If you have found yourself with skin tags (Sorry, boo), there are a few ways to get rid of them. Believe it or not, tea tree oil is one method. Mix a few drops of the oil with water, put it on a cotton ball, then apply directly to the skin tag. Over time, it will get darker and should just fall off in a couple weeks. I'd hate to be the lucky recipient that finds it, but whatevs — it works. You can also use dental floss or thread to cut off the base of the skin tag and basically rip that thing off. Ummm. I think I'll pass. While you do have these at-home options, I wouldn't do any of that myself; I'd definitely schedule an appointment with a trained professional. Because skintag removal is considered a "cosmetic procedure" it will cost you about $150 per visit. Skin tags won't grow back but they may sprout up in other areas. The good news is, they're harmless; they just look pretty gross.

BOTOX

If visible fine lines and wrinkles are your concern, Botox is one of the best treatments out there to combat the visible signs of aging. I know some people feel weird about injecting Botulism in their face but the results are too good to ignore. Basically, a wrinkle is the result of repetitive muscle movement and Botox is injected into those wrinkles to essentially paralyze the muscle that makes them. It's not cheap and the price will usually go by the area being treated, or by unit. It can cost anywhere from $10 to $20 per unit. Results can last anywhere from three to six months. It's the quickest way to look like you've had a year-long vacation but, depending on how many areas you have treated or units you need, it might cost you a pretty penny too.

DERMAL FILLERS

As we get older we lose the firmness in our skin. It starts to sag and loss of volume will be visible. Getting old blows. When this is your concern, fillers are the best option. Fillers can be used to replace fat on the face and also add volume and contour to the cheeks, chin, and lips. Most people are concerned with their nasolabial folds, which are the lines from the nose to the mouth. These can be very prominent on some people but with the help of a filler, might be completely erased.

Back in the day, I used some filler to make it look like I actually had cheekbones. I sort of liked it but not enough to keep doing it. It wears off in about six months to a year so if you try it and hate the result, at least it's not permanent. Usually people use one to two syringes per treatment. The usual cost per syringe is $450 to $600. If you don't need that much, sometimes you can buy half a syringe and use the other half at your next appointment. Hey, I like any bargain. What can I say?

These are just some of the amazing pro treatments out there. It takes a little research to find the right treatment for you but, with any of these options, as long as you go to a trained professional, you should be able to get some amazing results.

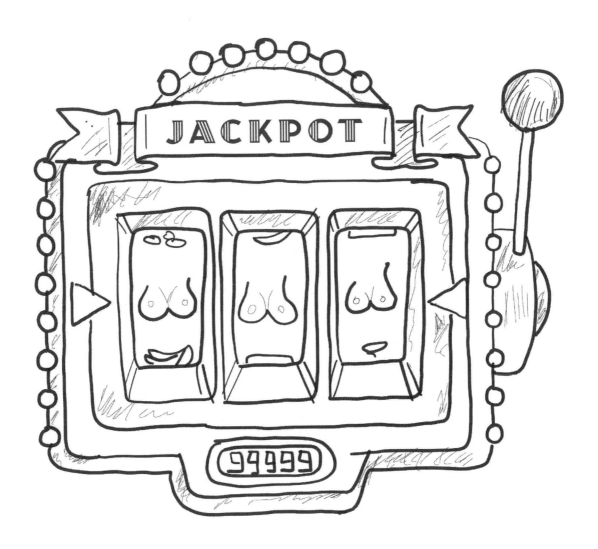

86

11

JACKPOT OF CANCER

MY JOB AS A BEAUTY TRAINER is to help people look their best. I find that when you look better, you'll usually feel better too. At your worst moments you might be tempted to give up on looking good — but sometimes all it takes is a little lipstick to make everything (almost) OK.

I was at work when I got the message. "If this is Jeremy Beth Michaels, can you please call me at this number as soon as you can?" That's the moment I knew: I had breast cancer. Having turned "a certain age," I had gone in for my first mammogram. The nurses warned me that if they found something, I'd have to come back to get a biopsy. However, they said that most of the time it's nothing and I shouldn't worry. Does silently panicking count as worry?

My neurotic anxiety proved to be well founded as they did find something, and I did have to go back. To date, the biopsy was the worst experience I've ever had in my life. I would rather get a root canal for 24 hours straight, without Novocain, while doing my taxes or putting something together from Ikea, than go through another biopsy. Let me explain the process for you: you disrobe, get on a table with a big hole in it for your breasts to be pulled through (Yes, I said pulled), then they sandwich them between two metal plates and stick a needle into your tit to withdraw the cells "in question" for examination. I was on that table for three horrifying hours.

I had two spots they needed to take a look at. As I sat on the table with only a local anesthetic to my breast, I could feel a vacuum going around and underneath the skin, followed by loud popping noises reminiscent of those packaging bubble sheets. Really pleasant. I laid there, tears rolling down my face because I couldn't compute this type of pain. After the procedure, I went home and sat catatonic for about two days, not really able to process — nor block out — what I had just experienced.

They ended up finding something questionable after the biopsy. I got ahold of the nurse on the phone and she told me, "Well, first of all, you got the jackpot of cancer. I mean, if you're going to get cancer, this is the one to get. It's called DCIS, which means it's enclosed and hasn't spread. You're really lucky." Wait, what? It only halfway registered in my brain. You just told me two words that should never be in the same sentence: jackpot and cancer.

They say timing is everything because that same week I got summoned for jury duty. That's like a double fuck you from the universe: I guess I was a total bitch in a past lifetime. But since I had to turn City Hall down because of my treatment, I've never been called up for duty again. Maybe they think I'm dead. So, there's at least one positive.

I guess I'm still in disbelief, even now, four years later. I know so many people who have also had cancer in various forms but they found out much later than me and ended up going through intense surgeries and months or years of chemotherapy sessions. My situation, I suppose, was rightfully considered a breeze. But it didn't feel that way to me. I felt ill, confused, and unsure of what would happen next. I was terrified during the entire treatment but I practiced my best Shakti Gawain and started visualizing the fuck out of everything positive.

After the biopsy, I met with the doctors in the oncology department to figure out the next steps in this fun journey. They said that my two and only two choices were a lumpectomy with radiation, or a mastectomy. Slim pickings. One choice sounded like an invitation to the worst party ever, while the other sounded like an invitation to the after-party to the worst party ever. Still, I had to go to at least one of them. All I knew was that I have a great rack. People pay good money for these things — I didn't want to lose 'em. So I told the doctors I didn't want to get all Angelina Jolie on them and get the drastic double mastectomy. I would stick to the other awesome option: the lumpectomy, in which they removed the abnormal tissue from my breasts.

I was scheduled to start the six weeks' radiation after I healed from the surgery. Radiation would be every day except Saturday and Sunday. (Hey, thanks so much for giving me the weekends off to party, guys!) Too bad that once I started treatment, I was so exhausted I couldn't stay awake past 8pm. For six weeks I sat in a waiting room with a bunch of other cancer patients and waited for my name to flash up on a screen. That's your cue to go in and get zapped. But somehow when I envisioned seeing my name in lights, it wasn't in the oncology department at Kaiser.

Of course now anything and everything to do with cancer was showing up all over the place: commercials, websites, articles, and Breast Cancer Awareness Month. Before this happened, I hadn't thought twice about cancer honestly. It just wasn't my reality. "It will never happen to me," I thought, as do so many women. And then when it does, you still can't believe it.

Everyone always says everything happens for a reason but how can you really justify getting cancer? Sometimes I think things just happen because they happen. There is no rhyme or reason but you create something to get through it and make it meaningful. I've been trying to do this since July 29, 2013, when I found out. I told myself that it probably means something amazing is going to happen in the future. I will get that dream job, that man (which I finally did! Thank you, Cupid), or win the lottery… You can tell yourself all sorts of affirmations, think positively, meditate, eat right, do yoga, get a crystal healing — but it doesn't change the fact you've been altered without your consent, forever. How do you get comfort in that? I'm still trying to figure it out.

I can't tell you how many strangers saw my breasts and I'm not talking about when I was cocktailing at my local waterhole, Ajax, in college. Frankly, those boob shows were for fun. Even when I went to New Orleans, at least I got beads for showing these beauts. (Me pointing to my boobs.) I felt like I brought Mardi Gras to Kaiser but when you undergo radiation you don't gets the beads. You get oddly placed, blue, pinprick-sized tattoos that mark where you've been radiated... and they definitely don't look as pretty or shiny.

Ironically enough, a few years ago when I was going through a rough breakup, I wandered into an amateur tattoo shop in Venice, California like an asshole and got a wishbone tattooed above my left breast. That's the one that got cancer: I guess I didn't make the right wish. So who do you call when you want to try and find some comfort? Obviously, your mom, right?

Well, my mom would inevitably say the wrong thing, even when she had the best intentions. I remember whenever I had broken up with a boyfriend, quit a horrible job, or got cancer, my mom would give me the same inane advice: "Just put on a little lipstick and everything will be OK." Now, I know it sounds shallow but as I've gotten older I really think there's something to this. It's the essence of the "fake it till you make it" mentality.

So when I got home after hearing I had freaking breast cancer, and that my life would forever be changed, I got out my favorite red lipstick. I put some on and looked in the mirror. Of course it didn't erase the fact I had gotten something that one in six people get but... it did make me look pretty, even if only on the outside — at least until my insides got pretty again too.

FOR A GOOD TIME FOLLOW:
@JEREMYTHEGIRL

MAKEUP TIP #11

THE PERFECT RED LIP TO MAKE EVERYTHING OK

WHAT YOU'LL NEED:

CONCEALER

LIP PENCIL

LIP BRUSH

LIPSTICK — PICK YOUR FAVORITE RED: MATTE, CREAMY, OR GLOSSY

CREAM OR POWDER HIGHLIGHTER

KLEENEX

TRANSLUCENT FINISHING POWDER

Make sure your lips are clean and dry. Get a little bit of concealer, gently brush it all over lips, and blend it into your lip line to prime and prepare your lips for lipstick. You don't need a lot, just enough to canvas your lip area. This will also fill in any fine lines and smooth out the surface of your lips. Next, get a lip pencil. You can use any color but if you're going for a bright red, a nude or red lip liner will work just fine. Trace your lip line with the pencil and then fill in your lips completely. If you want to make your lips bigger, here's your chance to extend a little past your actual lip line till you get your desired shape. Lining your lips will help your lipstick stay on all day and will also help guide you when you apply it, so you don't go outside the lines.

Now you can apply some lipstick onto your lip brush, which will give you more control than using the lipstick itself, and start filling in your lips. Starting from the center, go outwards until your lips are at your desired color. You can experiment with any color you want. Try new shades and the best part is, you can always wash it off if you don't like it. Once you've perfected your color, grab a Kleenex, fold it in half and gently blot your lips.

For a little drama you can draw attention to your Cupid's bow. Take a little cream or powder highlighter and blend it along this area to accentuate your lip line, giving you a sexy pout with minimal effort.

Nothing is more unattractive than having lipstick on your teeth so, to prevent this, take your pointer finger, put it in your mouth, and suck on your finger as you pull it out. (This is really great to do on first date by the way.) I realize it looks like you're performing something sexy on yourself, or for an audience if you're in public, but this is the only method I've found to make sure you don't look like a bag lady.

Finally, dust some translucent finishing powder gently on your lips and — congrats! — you've set your look. Just like me, you've put on a little lipstick and now everything will be OK. Even if it isn't, at least you look amazing and you got to give your finger a blowjob.

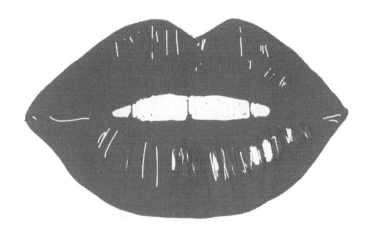

12

CAN YOU HEAR ME NOW?

CANCER ISN'T THE ONLY HURDLE I'VE OVERCOME; I was deaf until the age of seven due to a milk allergy. In order to find out exactly what I was allergic to, I had to have special allergy tests. One test I remember vividly was where they injected all these different things into my back, like a grid. It took hours. My friends and family could have used me for a tic-tac-toe board for days after that appointment.

Once the doctors figured out my allergies stemmed from lactose, and specifically milk, I was taken off any and all dairy products. Within a matter of weeks my sense of smell and hearing came back. Of course this was awesome, but it did mean my tiny silent world was about to become very pungent and loud. And that's NOT at all a confusing thing to happen to a little girl.

Years later my mom told me the story about how they figured out I had a problem: She was trying to get my attention one day by calling my name from across the room, but I didn't hear her. This went on for about 10 minutes and she was getting really irritated. Finally, she came over to me, turned my face towards hers, and yelled, "Why aren't you answering me, Jeremy

Beth?" (That's how you knew you were in real trouble if your mom used your WHOLE name.) And I told her, "You know I can't hear you, Mommy, unless you're looking at me."

There it was, I could only "hear" when I was looking directly at the person because I was reading their lips. And because I could talk fine, with none of the usual hearing impairment-type speech impediments, no one knew I had this disability. After the diagnosis, I had to go to a special learning center for the hearing impaired for about six months. I fucking hated it. We had to walk around with our eyes blindfolded; you'd hear random sets of claps and you had to walk to the beat across the floor. I do have a love of music and I love to dance so maybe the treatment is why I can do some epic body rolls when needed. (Believe me, there's a time and a place.) So, there's a plus right there.

We had recently moved from windy, cold Chicago to sunny, palm tree galore California. As I sat on our new back porch, looking out at our new glorious backyard, all the different scents had me hypnotized. Trees laden with olives and almonds. The juiciest, best tasting, strawberries I've ever had. And, at the center of the yard, roses in all different colors: yellow, peach, red, pink, white, burgundy, and orange. My dad would sweetly gather a vase full to put on the kitchen table whenever they were in multicolor bloom. They smelled so rich and sweet, I almost wanted to eat them. But I inhaled and stared with wonder instead.

There was an abundance of peaches, apples, apricots, plums, purple seedless grapes, lemons, and limes. I felt like I was living on a fruit stand. To add an even cooler factor, the trees surrounded a black-bottom pool that I spent half my youth in. Being able to smell a peach or a red rose for the first time was amazing when you'd gone your life up to that point scent deprived. Before I could smell, I used to draw people without any ears or a nose because, in my seven-year-old logic, if I couldn't smell or hear, neither could anyone else.

I loved my new aromatic world and it was also my first introduction to the world of beauty. That Christmas my mom gave me the best present ever: a perfume-making kit. The kit came with little, vintage-looking plastic bottles, dye to color the perfume, and essential oils of jasmine, rose, gardenia, lemon, and lime — all to experiment and create with. Once I was done making the perfect bouquet, I could design and label my fragrant creations. I played with this thing for months. I kept all my handcrafted perfumes on the windowsill like little trophies and they created colored prisms on my wall during the day.

When I wore the rose, I felt kind of empowered, strong, and feminine — or as much as you could when you're seven. The jasmine and gardenia scents made me think of summer picnics in the park and warm breezes. When I used lemon, lime, or any citrus, I found I was a little happier than usual. How is it possible that each scent made me feel differently? I knew early on I was onto something. Scents have a way of altering how we feel emotionally. Fragrance evokes memories, conjures up feelings, and can set your mood. It's just a matter of deciding what mood you're going for.

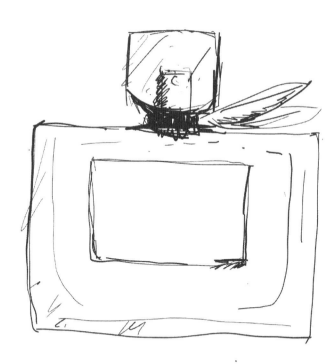

MAKEUP TIP #12

FINDING YOUR SIGNATURE SCENT

WHAT YOU'LL NEED:

YOUR NOSE

COFFEE BEANS

AN OPEN MIND

The best guide for wearing fragrances is: a little goes a long way. The basic rule is that you want your fragrance to be detected lightly if someone is standing in your personal space. If you leave a trail of really strong, overpowering fumes when you walk by, you're using waaaaaaay too much. And for real, don't wear fragrance to the gym. Just don't. It's bad enough when we have to smell someone's sweat while doing 60 minutes of Zumba. It's even worse when they're cloaked with heady patchouli before 9am.

Gauge your scent by the occasion but also take risks. A fragrance will react differently to each person's body chemistry so it may take some time to find your favorite signature scent. Most high-end retailers will have coffee beans to clear your sense of smell between sniffs so you can make sure you're getting an accurate read on your picks. Once you settle on your perfect scent, you'll be able to stink delicious all day and all night and hopefully you won't offend everyone around you.

Perfume creates a mood and a vibe; it can transport you to the future and can even bring back some long-forgotten memories. So when you're choosing a new fragrance, keep your mind open and let your intuition and emotions guide you. You might also find it helpful to read about the different intensities, forms, and notes, plus fragrance types for different occasions.

INTENSITIES

COLOGNE: Lightest strength. When you want a light veil of fragrance.

EAU DE TOILETTE: Medium strength. Will fade throughout the day.

PERFUME: Strongest strength. Will be the boldest and truest concentration of the scent.

FORMS

SPRAY: The most common form. Think of your favorite perfume bottle.

SOLID: Usually comes in a compact in balm form. You can apply this directly to pulse points on your wrists, behind the ears, neck, behind the knees. Really anywhere you'd like a soft fragrance to trail behind.

MIST: The lightest hint of fragrance. Perfect for any time you need a refresher, like happy hour after work or after a shower at the gym.

NOTES

THE TOP NOTES: The first scents you notice when you spray or apply to skin. Basically it's the first burst of fragrance you can detect. The top note lasts about thirty minutes to an hour. Usually citrus is the top note of fragrances because it lasts the least amount of time.

THE MIDDLE NOTES: Will last anywhere from one to three hours. It's the heart of the fragrance and will usually have floral notes, such as lavender or rose.

THE BASE NOTES: The main theme of the perfume. These will be the last notes of the fragrance you'll be able to notice after the top notes have evaporated. The base lasts three to five hours.

FRAGRANCE TYPES

FRESH/AQUATIC: Best scent for the workplace and during the day. Look for notes of bamboo, fresh cut grass, aquatic waters, and ocean sea salt. Aquatic notes are languid, ethereal and fresh. I like to wear these types of fragrances when I go to a day party, family function, or baby shower. Think freshly washed linens hanging from a clothesline, or a day at the beach.

FLORAL: Can go from day to night. Think Bulgarian rose, jasmine, lily-of-the-valley, tuberose, peony, and freesia. You can't go wrong wearing a floral on a first date, meeting the parents, or when you want to bring out your romantic, feminine side.

FRUITY: Best during the day. Think of any delectable fruit like coconut, cherries, blackberries, raspberries, pear, watermelon, peaches, and nectarines. Fruity fragrances can be quite strong but not in an overpowering way; they're like sprinkles of happiness on your skin. Wearing this type of scent is great for a summer party, or when you're about to go on an adventurous trip.

CITRUS: Think brunch or shopping with the girls. Scents with orange, lemon, limes and grapefruit work best when you need a pick me up after a long night, or when the rain is making you feel gloomy!

WARM AND SPICY: These scents are great for evenings, winter, and date nights. Patchouli, pepper, cinnamon, ginger, cardamom, nutmeg, coffee, and clove are fiery, bold and alluring, delivering a unique and tempting fragrance. Consider these your LRD — little red dress. This is where you throw out the basic black and step it up in boldness.

EARTHY AND WOODY: Day or night but has a sophisticated feel. Think board meeting. You have the lead role for the play or you're asking for a raise. Amber, cashmere, leather, mescal, pine, sandalwood, and cedar are some of the dominant notes. These scents are warm and kind of have a worn-in feel. Almost like playing in your dad's study.

GOURMAND: Sweet fragrances are best in the evening, winter or when you're about to have some sexy time. These are the most decadent of all the scents. Think molten chocolate cake, vanilla, hot chocolate, pound cake, brown sugar, and almond lattes. Wear these notes when you want to remember your childhood, you have a fondness for sweets, or you just want to smell edible.

FUN GROSS FACT: You remember when Lady Gaga was coming out with a perfume? Her scent, Fame, was rumored to smell like blood and semen. I don't even like that shit out of a body so why would I pay a hundred clams for a bottle of it? If someone ever gave it to me, I'd just give them po, po, po, poker face in Gaga's honor.

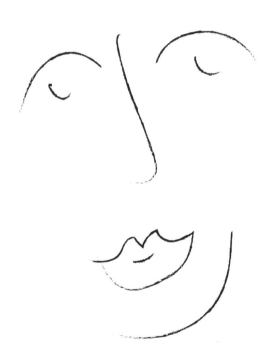

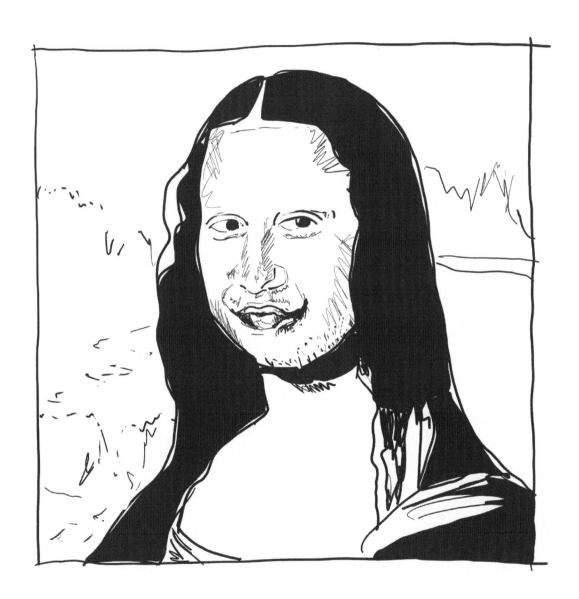

100

13

SELFIE NATION

I AM SAD TO SAY THIS IS AN ACTUAL CHAPTER. What kind of sick world do we live in where we spend more time perfecting our selfies than we do helping the needy? Every time someone takes a selfie a hot bowl of chicken noodle soup should appear in the hands of a starving person. But if you prefer to let people die of hunger, then at least let me give you the proper tools to slay every picture, every time. Lighting, filters: Hello, Kylie Jenner!

One thing I've noticed working in the beauty industry in LA over the years is all the bad cosmetic surgery. I should carry around before-and-after pictures of Kenny Rogers (Awww, poor thing) just to show my clients what can happen if things go south. You gotta know when to fold 'em!

Recently, I was working an event in Hollywood (a town no stranger to cosmetic "improvements") and a woman came in who was probably in her late forties. Her lips were so inflated they looked like inner tubes you'd see drifting on a lake during summer. Her mouth was even fuller than the famously coveted "Angelina Jolie pout." Equally as distracting were her breasts, which were practically resting on her collarbone, sticking straight out of nowhere and basically staring at me. Being garden gnome-sized myself, those things were eye level. So now I know why men can't take their eyes off of boobs: They're super distracting.

Oddly enough, this woman was only looking for black eyeliner. I wanted to kindly tell her that no one would ever be looking at her eyes as they'd be so fixated with her enormous teets and clownish lips. Quite frankly, I can't even remember if she had any eyes. She could have been wearing an eye patch and hobbling on a peg leg and no one would have even noticed her eyeless face. But still I helped her find an eyeliner and she was on her way. To this day, I can't remember her face but I remember her lips and boobs.

Don't get me wrong, I'm all for subtle enhancements — whether it be facials, a little Botox here, or a little filler there. But if you're going to get work done, you should want to look like a better version of yourself, not a caricature drawing you'd get at a shitty county fair by some old guy named Al who has one tooth left. You know, where he gives you an exaggerated chest and huge bee-stung lips while you're riding a Ferris wheel and smoking a corncob pipe. And seriously: if you're trying to go against the laws of physics, it's probably time to have a long conversation with yourself or get a mirror that lies (or at least one that has an adjustable, candlelit pink hue because every bitch looks amazing in candlelight).

All I know is, that lady got me thinking about our generation and I attribute some of this desire to be perfect nowadays to our access to instant communication. If you post a picture of yourself, you'll get positive and negative comments within minutes, even seconds. There's so much room for unwarranted criticism that it breeds massive insecurities. And while plastic surgery has been around for years, people didn't use to advertise it so promptly. They just went along their merry way and if you saw somcone who may have gotten some "work" done, you assumed they'd just had a really awesome four-day nap. On the other hand, if you saw someone who looked completely outrageous, with the huge inflated lips, the overblown cheeks, and the plumped-up face from too much filler, you weren't notified in a split second like today. And you definitely didn't see the minute by minute pictures of it flashing before your eyes in a news feed.

There's this insane access to immediate commentary from Instagram, Twitter, Snapchat, Facebook and all the other social media sites, yet whether it's positive or negative is up to the perceiver. Instant feedback perpetuates the need for women (or men) to compete and one-up each other by seeing who's the hottest, creating further unrealistic doubts and unattainable beauty standards. In turn, this begets the never-ending cycle of competition and it's basically pitting every woman (or man) against anybody in the world with a phone. Seriously, the only groups that are exempt are babies and dead people.

We see the current standard of beauty through magazines and social media, which convey a false reality in the sense that most pictures are "doctored," without the subject having to see an actual doctor. (By the way, the Vintage filter is always awesome! Try it.) We get bombarded with messages about what's "perfect." The perfect weight, the perfect breast size, and the perfect lips. How can we not want to change the way we look to fit that "perfect" mold? I succumb to it too. There are at least a couple days a week where I feel inferior: too fat, too old, and too short.

Of course, we all want to look our best at any stage of life, but at what point are these physical and photographic enhancements playing right into all of our fears about beauty, aging, and society? While it's important to feel good about ourselves externally, there's also a need for "internal enhancements" if you will: feeling good about your accomplishments, attaining your goals, or just not being an asshole are pretty cool features of a person too. They should put stuff like "10 Acts of Kindness You Can Do For Yourself That Don't Involve Your Looks" on the cover of Cosmo, not "How To Take That Perfect Selfie To Get Him Back."

But in an overly sexualized, youth- and beauty-centric culture, it's hard not to get sucked into wanting to alter the way we naturally look. Sure, if I could walk around looking like the finely filtered picture of myself at all times, I would. In the meantime, I'll keep doctoring up my own pics. As truly one of the most un-photogenic people of all time, I've learned a few tricks along the way and I can help you look your best, too, even if you're pretty ugly in real life. I'm kidding. I'm sure you're gorgeous — but we all need a little help from time to time.

MAKEUP TIP #13

APPS AND ANGLES TO GET THAT KILLER SHOT

WHAT YOU'LL NEED:
YOUR PHONE
ACCESS TO THE APP STORE
DOWNLOAD ANY OF THESE OR SEARCH FOR A FEW ON YOUR OWN:
BEAUTY PLUS (MY FAVORITE)
YOUCAM MAKEUP — MAGIC SELFIE MAKEOVERS
PERFECT365 — ONE-TAP MAKEOVER

OK, so check this out: When you want to get that effortlessly candid looking shot to post to all your social media sites, do what I do and spend some quality time with yourself. Get all primped to go absolutely nowhere but the comfort of your own home and spend the day on a fun, private modeling shoot. Put on some music, grab your favorite outfit(s), your favorite lipstick, and take a few shots of yourself.

For the best selfies, I like to hold my phone above my head with the phone aiming down so I can look up. It's naturally more pleasing to the eye than coming straight on. You also want to make sure you're in some natural light, which will give your skin healthy glow. I tilt my head from right to left, tilt my head down and then up, take several shots on both sides, and then pick the best ones.

Next, I perfect the pics with my chosen photo app. What's awesome is that you can put so many different types of filters on your pics. Filters have the ability to give your picture a totally different look and vibe. For instance, if you choose a filter with more of a golden glow, it will soften any picture, making it almost vintage and cozy looking. They can lighten, darken, add mystery, dimension, or whatever type of look you're going for. You can choose filters to enhance color or even make your pictures black and white.

You can do all sorts of fun enhancements to your face without having to spend $350 for a consult with your local plastic surgeon. You can smooth out your skin, if it doesn't look peaches-and-cream ready, with just a tap of your finger. You can make yourself look taller and thinner. (Honestly, I may never leave my house again. Oh, wait. The pizza is here, brb.) Yes, I said taller and thinner with one gentle swipe on your phone. You also can diminish dark circles, enlarge or brighten your eyes, and even remove acne if you're having a break out.

You are the Annie Leibovitz of your social media feed. Get creative, blow off eight hours of your life, and get thousands of pictures to post freely with confidence. Then you'll be, Hello, instant fans and followers! (and potential stalkers.)

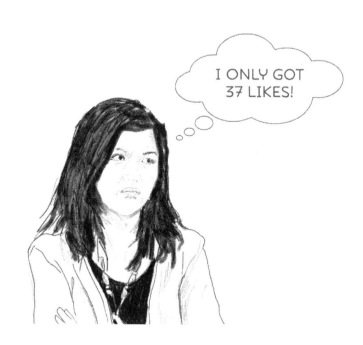

MAKEUP TIP #13B

FOUNDATION TYPES TO SLAY YOUR SELFIES

WHAT YOU'LL NEED TO DO:

CHOOSE WHERE YOU WANT TO BE ON A SCALE OF NATURAL TO PLASTIC

PICK THE RIGHT PRIMER FOR YOUR SKIN TYPE

PICK THE RIGHT FOUNDATION COVERAGE AND FINISH

GET YOUR SMILE READY!

Before you can point and click with precision, your foundation needs to be flawless.

You wouldn't paint a house without priming it, would you? So you need to do the same with your face. Primers help your makeup stay on all day, hide any discolorations, smooth out any rough texture, and provide a smooth surface for your foundation to glide over. Likewise, there are different types of foundation for different levels of coverage. To take the perfect selfie, you'll need to find out what type of coverage you want.

TYPES OF PRIMERS

HYDRATING AND ANTI-AGING: Putting makeup on overly dry skin makes you look older (and nobody wants that) because it seeps into all those crevices and valleys, which we in the biz call fine lines and wrinkles. By adding a moisturizing primer you automatically make your skin look more youthful and your makeup is way easier to apply.

COLOR CORRECTING: Acne scars, dark circles, and sallowness can all be adjusted here. Different color correctors do different things. You can use yellow or peach to counteract dark circles under the eyes or eyelids; green hides any redness to the skin; lavender will help banish a sallow complexion.

PORE MINIMIZING AND OIL CONTROL: Can you fry up some sizzling rice on your forehead? Do you hate the look of your pores? Do you feel like you're looking at the moon when you see the crater-like texture on your skin? Even if the texture of your skin looks and feels like a bag of twigs, using a pore-minimizing primer can smooth the roughest complexion and absorb any oil, making it super easy to follow with your foundation.

TYPES OF FOUNDATION COVERAGE

SHEER COVERAGE: Good for when you have five minutes to swipe something across your face, evening out your complexion so you look presentable to the outside world. My guess is you still wouldn't want to see your ex, but you could do so with less embarrassment than if you wore nothing at all.

MEDIUM COVERAGE: Perfect for day or night, it will cover any visible imperfections but you won't look too made up. You'll look polished and professional.

FULL COVERAGE: You could be sitting on top of a moving helicopter while it's flying and your makeup will stay put. Full-face coverage is like, Damnnnnn bitch, you literally spent at least two hours doing your makeup. Seriously, I can admire the art, but for most of us who aren't competing in a beauty pageant, it's just not practical for everyday. Still, if that's the way you wanna play, you go, girl. When I wear full coverage, it's usually because I have an all-day event and I don't want my look to budge.

DEWY FINISH: Can be sheer to full coverage. It provides a youthful luminosity to the skin, which is best for drier skin.

NATURAL FINISH: The "girl next door look" for your face. It almost looks like you don't have anything on but the joke is on everybody else because you do. Suckers!

MATTE AND SEMI-MATTE FINISH: The full-face look with little to no shine. Great for oilier skin types that want to look like they've never had one bead of sweat or oil on their forehead.

FINISHING POWDER/SETTING POWDER: You just put your makeup on, so why do you need a finishing powder to set your look? Think of it like hairspray but for your face: not a fleck of makeup will be out of place after a light dusting of powder.

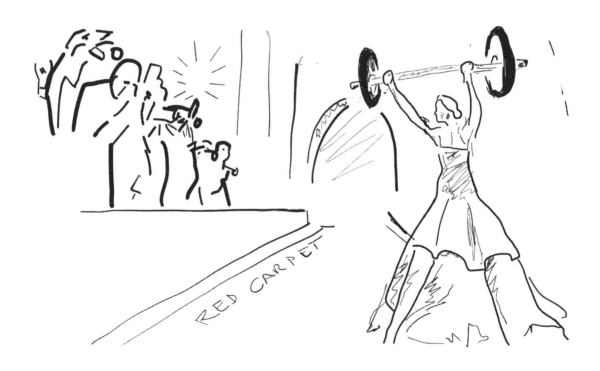

14

IT'S THE GYM, NOT THE RED CARPET

LADIES, FOR THE LOVE OF YOUR FAVORITE LIPSTICK, you're going to the gym, not a red-carpet event! Can we please calm down the pre-workout coiffing and perfuming?

No joke, I witnessed a girl at the gym wearing eyelash extensions that made Instagram and YouTube sensation @patrickstarrr look au naturel! With her platinum blonde hair extensions perfectly spiraled into beachy, just-fucked curls, she looked ridiculous as she lifted dumbbells up to her collar bone, squealing as she struggled to let them down in her tight as fuck, florescent pink outfit. She looked like a hooker who had just stumbled off Santa Monica Boulevard after a slow night — not one inch of her wasn't perfectly prepped for this trip, and this is just to workout? I'd be scared to see what her "Friday Night Club Look" would be. Homegirl, you're at the gym! You just got ready for four hours to get sweaty and it's not even 10am! To top it off, she was wearing the strongest musk perfume and I think I had a small asthma attack as she sashayed by in her Lululemon's.

Here's my question: Do you really think you're going to meet the man of your dreams at Club Sweat, Stank and Balls? Are you of the mindset that you have to look perfect at all times? At the grocery store? While getting the mail? While walking the dog? If so, you need to take it down a goddamn notch. As women, I know we're pressured to look photo ready at all times, but I'm giving you all permission to give yourself a pass from any primping before the gym. In fact, I insist on it!

Sometimes, I like to not get ready. I try and look as shitty as possible while at the gym and out running errands so then when I do finally get all cleaned up, people are actually surprised to see the finished product. And not to toot my horn, but I clean up pretty well. (Hi, boys!) Seriously, why would you waste your time and your foundation? You're there to work on your body, not your face. This is the one time of the day when you don't have to be concerned with how well you've contoured. So fucking enjoy it!.

Like every other woman, I spend half of my life getting ready. Don't you want a day off? I am definitely not going to get ready to get sweaty. It even sounds stupid to write. Working in the beauty industry, I have to don a full face of war paint everyday and my nails have to be perfectly dipped and tipped while I model and hock the latest makeup trend. So, honey, when I have a day off, I revel in it. You should too! C'mon, let's do it together!

There is a time and place for crimson red lips, but it's not when you're about to go into Orange Theory. Every minute beforehand does not need to be spent on trying to look runway ready. While I do believe in getting your body in the best possible shape, not everyone is built like Gigi Hadid or Emily Ratajkowski. (Fuck you guys, btw!) But we can at least try or dream, right? We all know about the benefits of endorphins that are released when you exercise, and which help to balance your mind, body, and spirit. Good health is truly one of the best cosmetics in the world: no one feels more beautiful than after a trip to the gym (unless you have three pounds of makeup dripping off your face).

Save your full makeup regimen for when you're out in the real world: for a date, a job interview, or a happy hour — not pumping iron on a Tuesday at 9am. Take it from me: No one cares how flawless your smoky eye is at the gym. Everyone is trying to burn off that last shitty plate of carbs they ate too.

MAKEUP TIP #14

LOW-KEY BEAUTY

WHAT YOU'LL NEED:

FACE WIPES

HYDRATING OR TINTED MOISTURIZER

MASCARA — IF YOU INSIST

SUNSCREEN

Let's make a pact that there should be no primping before pumping. The best way to prepare your face for the gym is to make sure your skin is clean and moisturized. When you work out, you want to keep your skin bare and without a stitch of makeup so your skin can breathe and sweat out toxins. This will help with clogged pores and breakouts, and also get rid of any unwanted debris left on the surface of your skin. None of that can happen when you're wearing a full face of makeup. But if you must primp a bit because you can't stand to see your bare face grimacing in the mirror as you do squats, then indulge in a basic tinted moisturizer and a light coat of mascara.

Personally, I like to use those handy face wipes you get at any drug store or high-end retailer. There are different types: exfoliating, purifying, hydrating, and for sensitive or acne-prone skin. I use them to clean my face before and after my workout. You'd be surprised at how much dirt is on your face that you can't see. Pretty gross, right? Trust me on this one. Once I've made a clean sweep and there's no filth visible on the wipes (usually takes one or two), I follow with a hydrating moisturizer because my face is always dry. But regardless of your skin type, it's important to keep your skin hydrated before and after sweating and losing fluids. Also, if you're going outside after your hour of cardio, please remember to put on sunscreen, or you can simply use a moisturizer that has sunscreen in it.

Stick to these basics and not only will you be pumped but you'll be primped just enough to work out those triceps. Or, dammit, your bingo wings. B-13!

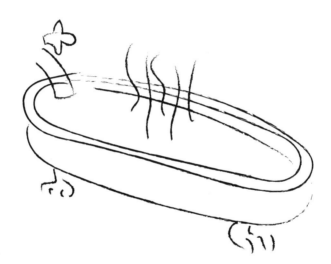

15

LIONS, TIGERS, AND FACEWIPES

ONE THING I'VE LEARNED OVER THE YEARS is that you can bring a little bit of glamour wherever you go… even if that wherever has bears, spiders, and cow shit. Yep, I'm referring to camping. Didn't think you'd find a chapter about camping in a makeup book, did ya? Never underestimate the power of beauty in a dirty situation.

Every year on the third weekend in June, I go on a lakeside camping/houseboat party. It's a great time with good friends, music, day drinking, laughter, dancing, and did I mention more dancing? You wouldn't think people could look fabulous traipsing through dung while sleeping in tents but it happens at what we call "LDP" (Lake Don Pedro). We camp and party on this huge hill with a few houseboats docked on the lake. It's usually a couple hundred of our closest friends. (Yes, I'm that popular.)

I'll admit I'm not the most avid camper. I like room service, hot bubble baths, and eight-hundred thread count Egyptian cotton sheets. This is not that kind of trip. For one thing, I had to get used to the communal outhouse, which you can imagine gets pretty sexy after a few days of people partying. Yum. Second is the sleeping situation. Being a camping novice, I bought a tent off the Internet that claimed it could sleep two people. I'm thinking it had to have been for a tiny elf, because remember I'm 4'11" and I barely fit in there myself. FYI, 4'7" is considered little-person height. So they should probably amend their description to say, "Fits two very little-sized people… uncomfortably."

Thanks to this annual trip, I've grown to love camping but I never felt totally comfortable until I saw my friend Melinda's Glam Camp. It was like being at home, or at least a really awesome ladies' boudoir. The best way to describe Melinda is pin-curl retro with a side of marvelous, fabulous, and a hint of this bitch slays all day. We call her Bender Barbie because when we get out on the lake, before she gets her unending drink on, she sets up a whole freakin' salon for our campsite. We have a lot of time on our hands so why not look pretty while swatting flies, throwing back cold ones, and laying in the sun?

Well, luckily for all the campers, there's no beauty item you can't find at Glam Camp. She brings ALL of her makeup. And I do mean all of her makeup. I'm talking about two train cases full of everything her fellow campers may need to get properly dressed up: anything from your low-key lady of leisure look to a wild outfit for our big Saturday night costume party. Maybe you need to sport an adhesive glitter bindi or a faux beauty mark for your ecstasy-dosing dusk rendezvous…

Melinda comes prepared with fifty of her makeup brushes, a full-length mirror, and one of those weird and disturbing close up mirrors that magnify everything. Truthfully, these mirrors are a cruel and unusual punishment under any circumstances, let alone on a camping trip when you haven't washed your face for days, and have passed out in the dirt for the previous few nights… that's if you've slept at all.

We have themed parties and she brings two dozen kinds of wigs and costumes in case Eighties Rocker is calling your name, or maybe a Fancy Streetwalker look is more your speed? Any look you're going for, she can emulate. She packs more glitter, hats, hair extensions, face masks, and nail polishes than all the contestants on RuPaul's Drag Race combined!

Just to give you a little peek into Melinda, she brings this booze called Damiana. It's a golden liquor in a bottle the shape of a fat sumo-wrestling woman. You don't really drink it; you shoot it. The myth behind Damiana is that it's supposed to help you get "ready for love." So when she gives us our shots, about every two hours (Hey, we like to party), she says, "Don't get pregnant." Luckily, I didn't.

I was amazed that she could walk up and down this steep, ninety-degree hill, with five-inch fuck me pumps on, and never fall down. With or without booze, this is a pretty impressive feat. Melinda made me realize you don't have to be going to a club or a photo shoot to look and feel glamorous. You can do it anytime, anyplace. Under her influence, I've never felt more beautiful in my life, while not showering for three days.

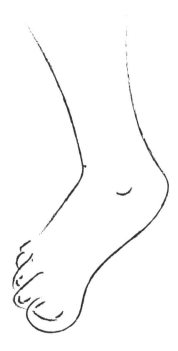

MAKEUP TIP #15

ESSENTIALS FOR GLAMPING AND THE GREAT OUTDOORS

WHAT YOU'LL NEED:
FACE WIPES

SPRAY FACIAL TONER

MOISTURIZING SUNSCREEN (AND OF COURSE YOUR EYE CREAM)

Sometimes after a long day of fishing and hunting I like to… Who am I kidding? After a long day of relaxing on the lake in a big blue floaty, getting tan, and drinking lots of adult beverages while being hit by incredibly warm breezes, you really want to keep your skin clean, hydrated, and protected from the sun. Alternately, if you ever find yourself stuck in the wild, out on the side of a road, or camping with your closest friends and you want to stay your freshest, take these few things and you'll be fine. I simply can't live without them.

Like for the gym, I always have a pack of ready-to-use facial wipes. I love these things because they're convenient and you can find them at almost any beauty retailer, plus they're great for any type of skin. They magically take off any traces of makeup and are refreshing, especially if you're getting wasted in the sun.

I also like to keep my skin hydrated during a day in the sun by spraying on a facial toner, which will keep your pores closed, shutting out wind-borne debris. I usually like to get a rose-water toner because it's hydrating, brightening, and anti-aging. Using a toner restores the balance in your skin. And because most toners also help to moisturize and soften the skin, they actually diminish fine lines and wrinkles by plumping them up. Toner is like your portable genie in a bottle and you definitely need it when you don't have showers around.

After I use my toner, I like to wait for it to soak in — usually about ten seconds — and then I follow with my moisturizing sunscreen. Sunscreen is potentially going to save you years of syringes of Botox down the road, while also protecting you from skin cancer, premature aging, and sun spots. By applying sunscreen, you can still feel like a devoted sun worshipper but not look like one. And have I mentioned eye cream in this book? Never forget it! Your eyes are the first to show visible signs of aging. Let's attempt to keep those lines at bay.

BONUS TIP: Perfume attracts bugs and therefore bug bites so lay off your fancy fragrances when camping. You might want to smell amazing but the downside is you'll probably have a whole swarm of bees following you. You know that saying, you attract more bees with honey? Well, don't be the honey, Honey.

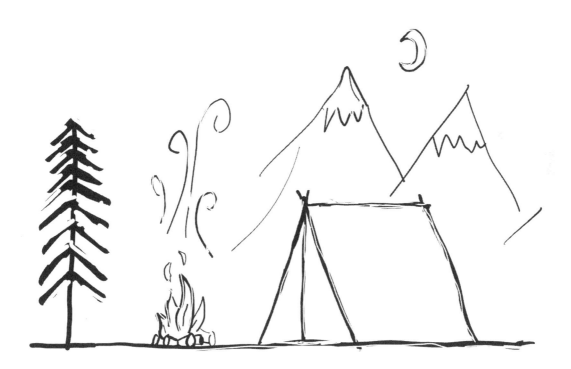

MIRROR, MIRROR

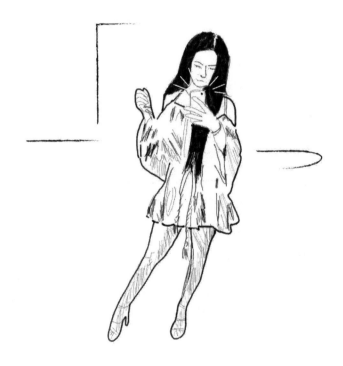

16

YOU LEFT THE HOUSE LOOKING LIKE THAT?

TIME AND AGAIN, CLIENTS AND FRIENDS ASK ME THE SAME QUESTIONS about what makeup to wear to certain events. But it's really just a matter of applying the same common sense that you would to clothes. Would you wear a pair of thigh-high black boots, an insanely skimpy skirt, and a tube top to a baby shower? Leather chaps with no pants to church? Are you sliding on some Lucite heels to go to your daughter's ballet recital? Probably not the vibe you want to go for. Likewise, it's best to consider the occasion before you break out that black lipstick. It never looks good at a PTA meeting — I tried.

That said, we live in a time where you can express yourself as much or as little as you want. Be yourself. Be unique. Seriously, if you want to be the only one at your stuffy cousin's wedding reception sporting a metallic green lip, go for it. I'd be impressed.

The aim of this book is to help clear up the confusion around beauty and to help you become your most beautiful self — whichever looks you prefer. One thing you should hear in the back of your mind when you finish reading this is: You're pretty. Just remember to keep your mind (and makeup bag) open.

MAKEUP TIP #16

LOOKS TO MAKE THE RIGHT IMPRESSION

WHAT YOU'LL NEED TO DO:
MIX AND MATCH ALL THE PRODUCTS AND TECHNIQUES IN THIS BOOK TO CREATE YOUR DESIRED EFFECT.

The following are my guidelines for some common events and situations. Hopefully these pearls of wisdom and a fine array of lipsticks will help you land that next job, get that second date, or look flawless on your wedding day.

JOB INTERVIEW

Maybe going with a navy blue lipstick isn't the best look when you're applying for a new corporate job. Focus more on your accomplishments and keep your look natural, fresh, and most importantly professional. Neutral tones work best. Now, if you're stripper looking to land a gig at SPEARMINT RHINO, that's a whole other set of tips and I think it involves more nipple tassels than mascara.

OFFICE WEAR/DAYTIME APPROPRIATE

Going simple but polished is your best bet. Keep it minimal. Keep your color palette neutral for the office. I like using browns, taupe, and greys. These colors are perfect for daytime. Tiffany in Finance can't focus on the books if she's too busy wondering how to copy your deep navy smoky eye.

HAPPY HOUR

This is when you can go from work to twerk. By using a couple extra coats of mascara and a touch up with your favorite dark eyeliner on your top lash line and your lower waterline, your look transitions from day to night. You can also add a little more drama by using a bright lipstick or a colored, ultra-shiny gloss to finish your look. Now you're ready for your two-for-one and hopefully you're not paying.

COCKTAIL PARTY

Guess what? You can add glitter even if you're over 13 and aren't going to a rave. Who doesn't like to sparkle every once in a while? It's all in how you apply it. For a cocktail party, you can add glitter, shimmer, or bold mattes: This is the one type of occasion where experimentation is expected and encouraged. Go for that bold red lip. Do that winged liner. What's stopping you? If you're using a highlighter, you can strobe that shit to the max. Focus on your brow bone, bridge of nose, Cupid's bow, and upper cheekbones for the ultimate glow.

Now there is a chance for overkill, so pick one feature you really want to play up and start from there. Usually, when I wear a smoky, glittery, or brightly shadowed eye, I'll pair it with a nude lip. I like to offset the boldness of my eyes with something subtle on the lips. Likewise, if I want to go for a bright lip, I won't go as heavy on the eyes. I'll go for something simple, like a lash-lined eye, either in black or dark brown, and a couple coats of mascara. If you want to get even fancier, you can add a pair of false eyelashes. The fun part is, you can go as intense or as blah as you want. At least now you have a starting point. Whatever look you're going for, make sure your bottles are getting popped!

FIRST DATE

Would you rather have your date focusing on the layers of your personality, or the layers of your foundation? First dates are tricky because you want to look hot, but not like so hot that you both are envisioning each other naked when you're drinking your first latte. My go-to look for a first date is simple, elegant, fun and flirty. Not too much foundation but enough to make your skin look amazing and dewy. A little bronzer and blush go a long way and help brighten up your overall complexion. For fun, you can add a bright color eye shadow or eyeliner to your upper lash line. You can do a small winged liner, which looks cute and flirty. Follow with a few coats of deep black mascara and top if off with a shiny, lip gloss. Now you'll look amazing and hopefully you're bypassing the awkwardness of any first date.

WEDDING DAY

Because this is the best day of your mom's life you don't want to look like shit during it. Make sure you get some word-of-mouth referrals for a great makeup artist, and definitely do a makeup trial before the big day so you can try out different styles. You want to look like the best version of yourself, not a creepy, overdone clown. I like to use neutrals, like different shades of muted browns, purples, peaches, and greys. But remember you can always add to your look, yet you can't take stuff away without washing everything off.

YACHT LIFE

Who cares? You're on a yacht. You win.

QUICK TREATMENTS BEFORE A SPECIAL EVENT

Now, this may sound really stupid but I've seen it time and again: Don't get a major chemical peel, or dramatically change your haircut, if you have an upcoming, important event. You can definitely use eye patches, energizing masks, and teeth whitening strips as great, easy add-ons to prepare for any special occasion. I like to do a hydrating or oxygen mask because it plumps and rejuvenates the skin, making it look fresh and firm. What more could you want? While I'm doing that I usually put on some teeth whitening strips. After about a half hour, my smile can brighten even the darkest day and my face looks as plump as a newborn baby's bum. I'm PageSix ready, everybody. Hey, we all are.

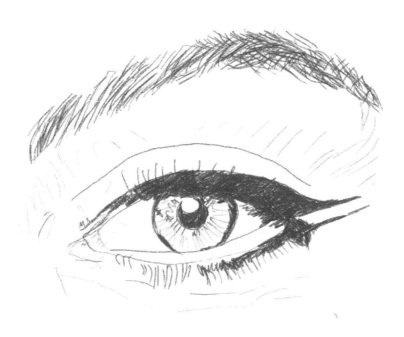

MAKEUP TOOL BOX

BEAUTY BLENDER: Why do I need to spend $20 on a sponge that doesn't even prevent pregnancy? I know, I ask myself this too. To use the sponge correctly, you need to wet it and then wring out any excess water. Then you can use it to apply your foundation in bouncing, pressing motions. This gives an incredibly airbrushed look, which is perfect for photos or when you want that flawless finish.

BRUSHES: Picasso didn't use his fingers to paint his masterpieces and neither should you. (Actually, sometimes he did. — ed.) Getting a decent brush set will help you perfect your makeup look. I only use synthetic hair for brushes. They're easy to clean, no animals are harmed in the process and they don't fall apart after three uses. You can find a good quality brush set at your favorite beauty retailer, usually for between $60 to $300. The main brushes you'll need are: all over face, flat foundation, blush, and eye shadow; flat or tapered flat edged brush, a crease or blending brush, and an eyeliner and a smudge brush to complete a full face confidently.

FACE WIPES: Hey, I'm lazy. Can't I just take off my makeup in bed? Now you can. Choose the wipes for your particular skin type.

Q-TIPS: Little cotton wonders on a tiny stick are proof of God's existence. What can't I do with these things? With a little water you can erase and correct any mistake. You need these in your makeup bag.

TWEEZERS: Nothing is sexier than seeing a long, thick, black wiry hair coming out of some place it's not supposed to. Make sure you always have these handy; you can even keep them in your car. Sunlight doesn't lie. Nothing is worse than going out for the day and catching a glimpse of this hair coming out of your face and you have nothing to remove it. Tweezers are also perfect for brow touch ups when you find a stray hair popping out of nowhere.

GLOSSARY OF TREATMENTS AND INGREDIENTS

All these treatments and ingredients will majorly increase your chances of attaining that "peaches and cream" looking complexion (even if we also have to use makeup to fake it). Talk to your friends, or a beauty expert; research different brands that peak your interest, and see what's new on the market. You can also read some reviews and blogs and if you want to believe all those "Influencers" out there these days, that's fine too. But the best thing is to try a product yourself and see what works best for you.

ALPHA-HYDROXY ACID: An exfoliating acid made from sugar cane that resurfaces the skin. Mostly recommended for dry skin. Also known as glycolic acid.

BIOTIN (VITAMIN B7): helps hair and nails grow. So what if you need to take four billion milligrams, this stuff really does work to keep your claws and mane growing at an unbelievable rate. A lot of hair products have biotin in them, which does help, but to get the best results you really have to take it internally.

BOTOX: If you can't get or afford Botox, you can use products to mimic the effects and look completely frozen in time. Look for ingredients like peptides, neuro-peptides, hyaluronic acid, and caffeine. These ingredients will plump, tighten, and firm the skin.

EXFOLIATION: You can exfoliate two ways: chemical (with an acid or enzyme) or manually (with beads). Both reveal newer, fresher skin. It's important to do this at least a couple times a week. Your skin care will work better and it will also help to eliminate the appearance of fine lines and wrinkles.

HYALURONIC ACID: This supreme hydrator attracts and retains up to 1,000 times its weight in water. Skin will look more supple and firm. It helps diminish the appearance of fine lines and wrinkles and keeps skin hydrated. This ingredient is great for both oily and drier skin types.

NIGHTTIME TREATMENTS: At night your body is regenerating itself so it's good to use something a little more potent at bedtime to renew all those deteriorating cells. Using a sleeping mask can help you get that skin you want. I absolutely love sleep masks because I am a lazy piece of crap. I can just slather one on and go off to dreamland, knowing I will wake up even prettier.

PEELS: Chemical or enzymatic peels can diminish fine lines, brighten uneven skin tones, remove sunspots and acne scars, and reveal younger looking skin. Only a fool wouldn't want that. You can get these at any makeup retailer these days. Enzymatic peels are usually better for sensitive skin, yielding almost the same results as an over the counter chemical peel.

PLASTIC SURGERY: Should I do it? How young is too young to get work done? This is a personal choice but remember you want to look like the best version of yourself, not a caricature. Some enhancements can't be corrected so really make sure you want to go under the knife. I recommend starting with a few fillers, which dissolve over a few months.

RETINOLS: Also known as Vitamin A, Retinol will help minimize fine lines, rough texture and uneven skin tone. It's like time in a bottle, when you don't have a lot of time left but you still want to look hot. For the best results, I usually suggest using a Vitamin C (to brighten and even out your skin) during the day and Retinols (to exfoliate and help with texture) at night — especially because retinols may make your skin sensitive to sunlight.

SALICYLIC ACID: An exfoliating acid made from willow bark, used in acne products. Mostly recommended for oily skin. This ingredient is able to clean out clogged pores and blackheads, and reduce sebum. Also known as beta-hydroxyl acid. Retinols may make your skin sensitive to sunlight so products are best used at night.

SERUMS: What the hell do they do and why do I need one? Why are they so expensive? Are there emerald cut diamonds in there for that price? Can't I just use Vaseline? Serums are the gateway to awesome skin and will usually cost a pretty penny. If you're going to drop some serious cash on yourself, here's where you want to do it. The consistency of serums are usually thinner and more watery than creams, so they have the ability to really soak into the skin, letting you absorb all the wonderful benefits of the product. Look for serums that combat whatever your skin concern is. For me, it's usually dehydration and fine lines. In that case, I'll pick something with hyaluronic or glycolic acid. It just depends on what my skin needs.

VITAMIN C: Brightens the skin and boosts your collagen and elastin. If you are concerned with aging, this is the ingredient I suggest using first. Not only does this ingredient fight free radicals it also helps to firm and tone, as well as eliminate fine lines and wrinkles. The only thing Vitamin C doesn't do is give you a back rub.

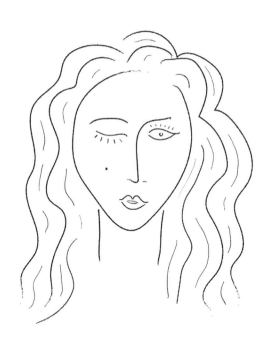

FOR A GOOD TIME FOLLOW:
@JEREMYTHEGIRL

ACKNOWLEDGEMENTS

"The best color in the whole world is the one that looks best on you."

— COCO CHANEL

Here's a list of people who believed in me, my unconventional beauty book, and encouraged me to never give up. For them, I am forever grateful.

My brother Joshie, for being the best brother a girl could ever ask for. Thank you for your genius artistic talents. This book couldn't have happened without you.

My editor, Elizabeth Allan, who took a de-railed train and helped, put it on the right track. Your talents don't go unnoticed. Free beauty advice for life!

My Mom and Dad, Thank you for being the coolest and most supportive parents in the whole wide world.

My true blue friend Amy Dresner, thank you for believing in me. It means more than you'll ever know.

My friend Jeff Kreisler, who still takes my calls and always reminds me to look up.

My friend Shelby Stockton, who never got sick of hearing about this book and cheered me on every step of the way.

My friend Steve Kassijikian, who laughs at all my jokes and appreciates my inappropriateness.

My PTR Family, who taught me how to properly take care of my skin and now I can pass the knowledge on.

My besties, April Annarino, Christina Morello, Lindsay Taylor, and Susie Marshall – I did it! Body roll to that.

My friend Shawn Pelofsky, who told me I could do it and I finally believe her. #clowntown forever.

All my clients (even the annoying ones), friends, and family who call asking for beauty advice without you, there would be no book. Thank you.

All my Sephora and Ulta cast and staff, thank you for giving me so much material all these years. You're all gorgeous!

And finally, my husband Matt, who listened to me talk endlessly about lipstick, blush, and skincare for the last four years and doesn't want to divorce me. I'm a lucky girl.